**ELSEVIER**

1600 John F. Kennedy Boulevard • Suite 1800 • Philadelphia, Pennsylvania, 19103-2899

http://www.theclinics.com

**PET CLINICS Volume 9, Number 1**
**January 2014 ISSN 1556-8598, ISBN-13: 978-0-323-26404-4**

Publisher: Adrianne Brigido
Developmental Editor: Susan Showalter

*PET Clinics* (ISSN 1556-8598) is published quarterly by Elsevier Inc., 360 Park Avenue South, New York, NY 10010-1710. Months of issue are January, April, July, and October. Periodicals postage paid at New York, NY, and additional mailing offices. Subscription prices per year are $225.00 (US individuals), $327.00 (US institutions), $115.00 (US students), $255.00 (Canadian individuals), $369.00 (Canadian institutions), $140.00 (Canadian students), $275.00 (foreign individuals), $369.00 (foreign institutions), and $140.00 (foreign students). To receive student and resident rate, orders must be accompanied by name of affiliated institution, date of term, and the signature of program/residency coordinator on institution letterhead. Orders will be billed at individual rate until proof of status is received. Foreign air speed delivery is included in all Clinics subscription prices. All prices are subject to change without notice. POSTMASTER: Send address changes to PET Clinics, Elsevier Health Sciences Division, Subscription Customer Service, 3251 Riverport Lane, Maryland Heights, MO 63043. **Customer Service: 1-800-654-2452 (U.S. and Canada); 314-447-8871 (outside U.S. and Canada). Fax: 314-447-8029. E-mail: journalscustomerservice-usa@elsevier.com (for print support); journalsonlinesupport-usa@elsevier.com (for online support).**

*Reprints.* For copies of 100 or more of articles in this publication, please contact the Commercial Reprints Department, Elsevier Inc., 360 Park Avenue South, New York, NY 10010-1710. Tel.: 212-633-3874; Fax: 212-633-3820; E-mail: reprints@elsevier.com.

Printed in the United States of America.

# Contributors

## CONSULTING EDITOR

**ABASS ALAVI, MD, PhD (Hon), DSc (Hon)**
Professor of Radiology, Division of Nuclear
Medicine, Department of Radiology, University
of Pennsylvania School of Medicine, Hospital
of the University of Pennsylvania, Pennsylvania
University, Philadelphia, Pennsylvania

## EDITORS

**STEFANO FANTI, MD**
Associate Professor, Director, Institute of
Nuclear Medicine, S.Orsola-Malpighi
University Hospital, University of Bologna, Italy

**CRISTINA NANNI, MD**
Consultant, Institute of Nuclear Medicine,
Policlinico S. Orsola-Malpighi University
Hospital, University of Bologna, Italy

**RICHARD P. BAUM, MD, PhD**
Chairman and Clinical Director, Professor
of Nuclear Medicine, Theranostics Center
for Molecular Radiotherapy and Molecular
Imaging, ENETS Center of Excellence,
Zentralklinik Bad Berka, Bad Berka, Germany

## AUTHORS

**ABASS ALAVI, MD, PhD (Hon), DSc (Hon)**
Professor of Radiology, Division of Nuclear
Medicine, Department of Radiology, University
of Pennsylvania School of Medicine, Hospital
of the University of Pennsylvania, University of
Pennsylvania, Philadelphia, Pennsylvania

**VALENTINA AMBROSINI, MD, PhD**
Nuclear Medicine, S.Orsola-Malpighi
University Hospital, University of Bologna,
Bologna, Italy

**RICHARD P. BAUM, MD, PhD**
Chairman and Clinical Director, Professor
of Nuclear Medicine, THERANOSTICS Center
for Molecular Radiotherapy and Molecular
Imaging, ENETS Center of Excellence,
Zentralklinik Bad Berka, Bad Berka, Germany

**MATTHIAS BLAICKNER, PhD**
Health & Environment Department, Biomedical
Systems, AIT Austrian Institute of Technology,
Vienna, Austria

**LISA BODEI, MD, PhD**
Deputy Director, Division of Nuclear Medicine,
European Institute of Oncology, Milan, Italy

**OTTO BOERMAN, PhD**
Department of Nuclear Medicine, Radboud
University Nijmegen Medical Centre,
Nijmegen, The Netherlands

**JAMSHED BOMANJI, MBBS, PhD, FRCR,
FRCP**
Head of Clinical Department, Consultant
Physician/Honorary Senior Lecturer, Institute
of Nuclear Medicine, University College
London Hospitals NHS Trust, London,
United Kingdom

**EMILIO BOMBARDIERI, MD**
Department of Nuclear Medicine, National
Cancer Institute, Milan, Italy

**MAARTEN BROM, PhD**
Department of Nuclear Medicine, Radboud
University Nijmegen Medical Centre,
Nijmegen, The Netherlands

**ARTURO CHITI, MD**
Department of Nuclear Medicine, Humanitas
Clinical and Research Institute, Milan, Italy

**MARTA CREMONESI, PhD**
Director, Division of Medical Physics,
European Institute of Oncology, Milan, Italy

**STEFANO FANTI, MD**
Associate Professor, Director, Institute of
Nuclear Medicine, S.Orsola-Malpighi
University Hospital, University of Bologna,
Bologna, Italy

**SARITA FORSBACK, PhD**
Turku PET Centre, Turku University Hospital,
Turku, Finland

**ANDOR W.J.M. GLAUDEMANS, MD**
Department of Nuclear Medicine and
Molecular Imaging, University Medical Center
Groningen, University of Groningen,
Groningen, The Netherlands

**MARTIN GOTTHARDT, MD, PhD**
Department of Nuclear Medicine, Radboud
University Nijmegen Medical Centre,
Nijmegen, The Netherlands

**SAILA KAUHANEN, MD**
Division of Digestive Surgery and Urology,
Turku University Hospital, Turku, Finland

**SELLAM KARUNANITHI, MD**
Department of Nuclear Medicine, All India
Institute of Medical Sciences, New Delhi, India

**JUKKA KEMPPAINEN, MD**
Turku PET Centre, Turku University Hospital;
Department of Clinical Physiology and Nuclear
Medicine, Turku University Hospital, Turku,
Finland

**KLAAS PIETER KOOPMANS, MD, PhD**
Department of Radiology and Nuclear
Medicine, Martini Hospital Groningen,
Groningen, The Netherlands

**HARSHAD R. KULKARNI, MD**
THERANOSTICS Center for Molecular
Radiotherapy and Molecular Imaging, ENETS
Center of Excellence, Zentralklinik Bad Berka,
Bad Berka, Germany

**RAKESH KUMAR, MD, PhD**
Department of Nuclear Medicine,
All India Institute of Medical Sciences,
New Delhi, India

**ALICE LORENZONI, MD**
Department of Nuclear Medicine, National
Cancer Institute, Milan, Italy

**ANNA MARGHERITA MAFFIONE, MD**
PET Unit, Department of Nuclear Medicine,
Santa Maria della Misericordia Hospital,
Rovigo, Italy

**HEIKKI MINN, MD**
Department of Oncology and Radiotherapy,
Turku University Hospital; Turku PET
Centre, Turku University Hospital, Turku,
Finland

**WIM J.G. OYEN, MD, PhD**
Department of Nuclear Medicine, Radboud
University Nijmegen Medical Centre,
Nijmegen, The Netherlands

**GIOVANNI PAGANELLI, MD**
Director, Division of Nuclear Medicine,
European Institute of Oncology, Milan, Italy

**EMMANOUIL PANAGIOTIDIS, MD, MSc**
Clinical Fellow, Institute of Nuclear Medicine,
University College London Hospitals NHS
Trust, London, United Kingdom

**GIOVANNA PEPE, MD**
Department of Nuclear Medicine,
Humanitas Clinical and Research Institute,
Milan, Italy

**DOMENICO RUBELLO, MD**
Director, PET Unit, Department of Nuclear
Medicine, Santa Maria della Misericordia
Hospital, Rovigo, Italy

**MARKO SEPPÄNEN, MD**
Turku PET Centre, Turku University Hospital;
Department of Clinical Physiology and Nuclear
Medicine, Turku University Hospital, Turku,
Finland

# Contents

Anna Margherita Maffione, Sellam Karunanithi, Rakesh Kumar, Domenico Rubello, and Abass Alavi

Novel diagnostic tools and therapies have emerged as a result of the continuous endeavors relating to neuroendocrine tumors (NETs). Nuclear medicine plays a pivotal role in the imaging and treatment of NETs. Somatostatin receptor analogues and metaiodobenzylguanidine remain front-line single-photon emission computed tomography (SPECT) radiotracers in the imaging of NET; their utility has been augmented by the increasing availability of SPECT/CT. Positron emission tomography has been growing rapidly in the imaging of NETs, paralleled by great efforts toward the development of new tracers. Hybrid imaging will play an important role in the future of NETs.

Giovanna Pepe, Emilio Bombardieri, Alice Lorenzoni, and Arturo Chiti

Different imaging strategies have been developed targeting the peculiar features of neuroendocrine tumors (NETs). Metabolic characteristics and receptor expression on the tumor surface have been studied, and expertise and knowledge are increasing as a result of the implementation of fusion imaging and the development of more detailed positron emission tomography tracers. Scintigraphic study of NETs is the most diffused and convenient technique for evaluating patients suspected to have NETs.

Heikki Minn, Jukka Kemppainen, Saila Kauhanen, Sarita Forsback, and Marko Seppänen

$^{18}$F-Fluorodihydroxyphenylalanine (FDOPA) is a powerful tool for the diagnosis and detection of neuroendocrine tumors when planning and monitoring surgical and oncologic therapies. Pheochromocytomas, paragangliomas, and medullary thyroid cancers especially are amenable to FDOPA imaging because of the high specific uptake of this amino acid analogue and excellent tumor-to-background contrast on PET/computed tomography.

Valentina Ambrosini and Stefano Fanti

$^{68}$Ga-DOTA-peptides are increasingly used for the detection of neuroendocrine tumors (NET) in clinical trials in Europe. They have been proved accurate for the detection of NET lesions (at primary and metastatic sites) and no adverse effects were recorded. Moreover, providing data on somatostatin receptors expression on NET cells, $^{68}$Ga-DOTA-peptides PET/CT is becoming a fundamental procedure to be performed before starting therapy and to guide treatment with either hot or cold somatostatin analogues. The easy and economic synthesis process is another advantage that is supporting its clinical use even in centers without an on-site cyclotron.

overexpress somatostatin receptors (SSTRs), which enable the diagnosis using radiolabeled somatostatin analogues. Internalization and retention within the tumor cell are important for peptide receptor radionuclide therapy. Use of the same DOTA-peptide for SSTR PET/CT using $^{68}$Ga and for peptide receptor radionuclide therapy using therapeutic radionuclides like $^{177}$Lu and $^{90}$Y offers a unique theranostic advantage.

Peptide receptor radionuclide therapy involves selective targeting of neuroendocrine tumors through somatostatin receptors with the aim to increase radiation dose to the tumors and spare normal tissue. The advantage of this internal radiation therapy is the ability to selectively target multiple metastases throughout the body. Early and accurate assessment of therapy response helps not only to identify the poor responders but also to personalize the treatment regimes with the aim of achieving maximum treatment benefit. This is the basis of theranostics.

Personalized dosimetry in radionuclide therapy has gained much attention in recent years. This attention has also an impact on peptide receptor radionuclide therapy (PRRT). This article reviews the PET-based imaging techniques that can be used for pretherapeutic prediction of doses in PRRT. More specifically the usage of $^{86}$Y, $^{90}$Y, $^{68}$Ga, and $^{44}$Sc are discussed: their characteristics for PET acquisition, the available peptides for labeling, the specifics of the imaging protocols, and the experiences gained from phantom and clinical studies. These techniques are evaluated with regard to their usefulness for dosimetry predictions in PRRT, and future perspectives are discussed.

# PET CLINICS

## PROGRAM OBJECTIVE

The goal of the PET Clinics is to keep practicing radiologists and radiology residents up to date with current clinical practice inpositron emission tomography by providing timely articles reviewing the state of the art in patient care.

## TARGET AUDIENCE

Practicing radiologists, radiology residents,and other health care professionals who provide patient care utilizing radiologic findings.

## LEARNING OBJECTIVES

Upon completion of this activity, participants will be able to:
1. Review nuclear medicine procedures in the diagnosis of neuroendocrine tumors including the use of 68Ga-DOTA-peptides, F-luorodihydroxyphenylalanine , SPECT tracers and PET tracers.
2. Discuss preclinical studies of SPECT and PET tracers for NET.
3. Describe patient selection for personalized peptide receptor radionuclide therapy using Ga-68 somatostatin receptor PET/CT, theranostics with Ga-68 somatostatin receptor PET/CT, and yttrium-based therapy of neuroendocrine tumors.

## ACCREDITATION

The Elsevier Office of Continuing Medical Education (EOCME) is accredited by the Accreditation Council for Continuing Medical Education (ACCME) to provide continuing medical education for physicians.

The EOCME designates this enduringmaterial for a maximum of 15 *AMA PRA Category 1 Credit*(s)™. Physicians should claim only the credit commensurate with the extent of their participation in the activity.

All other health care professionals requesting continuing education credit for this enduring material will be issued a certificate of participation.

## DISCLOSURE OF CONFLICTS OF INTEREST

The EOCME assesses conflict of interest with its instructors, faculty, planners, and other individuals who are in a position to control the content of CME activities. All relevant conflicts of interest that are identified are thoroughly vetted by EOCME for fair balance, scientific objectivity, and patient care recommendations. EOCME is committed to providing its learners with CME activities that promote improvements or quality in healthcare and not a specific proprietary business or a commercial interest.

**The planning committee, staff, authors and editors listed below have identified no financial relationships or relationships to products or devices they or their spouse/life partner have with commercial interest related to the content of this CME activity:**
Abass Alavi, MD, PhD (Hon), DSc (Hon); Valentina Ambrosini, MD, PhD; Richard P. Baum, MD, PhD; Lisa Bodei, MD, PhD; Otto Boerman, PhD; Jamshed Bomanji, MD, PhD, FRCP(Lond); Emilio Bombardieri, MD; Adrianne Brigido; Maarten Brom, PhD; Arturo Chiti, MD; Marta Cremonesi, PhD; Stefano Fanti, MD; Sarita Forsback, PhD; Andor W.J.M. Glaudemans, MD; Martin Gotthardt, MD, PhD; Kristen Helm; Brynne Hunter; Sellam Karunanithi, MD; Saila Kauhanen, MD; Jukka Kemppainen, MD; Klaas Pieter Koopmans, MD, PhD; Harshad R. Kulkarni, MD; Rakesh Kumar, MD, PhD; Sandy Lavery; Alice Lorenzoni, MD; Anna Margherita Maffione, MD; Jill McNair; Heikki Minn, MD, PhD; Cristina Nanni, MD; Mahalakshmi Narayanan; Wim J.G. Oyen, MD, PhD; Giovanni Paganelli, MD; Emmanouil Panagiotidis, MD, MSc; Giovanna Pepe, MD; Domenico Rubello, MD; Marko Seppänen, MD.

**The planning committee, staff, authors and editors listed below have identified financial relationships or relationships to products or devices they or their spouse/life partner have with commercial interest related to the content of this CME activity:**
Matthias Blaickner, PhD is a consultant/advisor for Phillips Austria.

## UNAPPROVED/OFF-LABEL USE DISCLOSURE

The EOCME requires CME faculty to disclose to the participants:
1. When products or procedures being discussed are off-label, unlabelled, experimental, and/or investigational (not US Food and Drug Administration (FDA) approved); and
2. Any limitations on the information presented, such as data that are preliminary or that represent ongoing research, interim analyses, and/or unsupported opinions. Faculty may discuss information about pharmaceutical agents that is outside of FDA-approved labelling. This information is intended solely for CME and is not intended to promote off-label use of these medications. If you have any questions, contact the medical affairs department of the manufacturer for the most recent prescribing information.

## TO ENROLL

To enroll in the PET Clinics Continuing Medical Education program, call customer service at 1-800-654-2452 or sign up online at http://www.theclinics.com/home/cme. The CME program is available to subscribers for an additional annual fee of USD 126.

## METHOD OF PARTICIPATION

In order to claim credit, participants must complete the following:
1. Complete enrolment as indicated above.
2. Read the activity.
3. Complete the CME Test and Evaluation. Participants must achieve a score of 70% on the test. All CME Tests and Evaluations must be completed online.

## CME INQUIRIES/SPECIAL NEEDS

For all CME inquiries or special needs, please contact elsevierCME@elsevier.com.

# Section I: Nuclear Medicine in the Diagnosis and Treatment of Neuroendocrine Neoplasms

# Nuclear Medicine Procedures in the Diagnosis of NET
## A Historical Perspective

Anna Margherita Maffione, MD[a], Sellam Karunanithi, MD[b],
Rakesh Kumar, MD, PhD[b], Domenico Rubello, MD[a],*,
Abass Alavi, MD[c]

## KEYWORDS

- Neuroendocrine tumor • Nuclear medicine • Imaging • Treatment • Therapy • PET • SPECT

## KEY POINTS

- In the last several years, novel diagnostic tools and therapies have emerged as a substantial result of the continuous endeavors relating to neuroendocrine tumors (NETs).
- Nuclear medicine plays a pivotal role in the imaging and treatment of NETs.
- Somatostatin receptor analogues and metaiodobenzylguanidine remain front-line single-photon emission computed tomography (SPECT) radiotracers in the imaging of NET; their utility has been augmented in recent years by the increasing availability of SPECT/CT.
- Positron emission tomography (PET) has been growing rapidly in the imaging of NETs, paralleled by great efforts toward the development of new tracers.
- Hybrid imaging, such as PET/CT or PET/magnetic resonance imaging, will play an important role in the future of NETs.

## NEUROENDOCRINE TUMORS: A CLINICAL POINT OF VIEW
### Pathologic Setting

Originally, the concept of neuroendocrine neoplasm reflected the hypothesis that the cells from which these tumors result from originated from the embryonic neural crest. This concept was invalidated years ago, but the term *neuroendocrine tumor* (NET) is still recommended by the World Health Organization's (WHO) most recent edition of the *WHO Classification of Tumours of the Digestive System*.[1]

During the last decades, multiple classifications for NET were proposed; as a result, divergences and confusions inevitably emerged, reducing the quality of the reporting data. In the last years, novel diagnostic tools and therapies have emerged as a substantial result of the continuous endeavors on this specific topic. The need for international standards has inexorably arisen. As a consequence, the International Union Against Cancer, the American Joint Cancer Committee, the WHO, and the European Neuroendocrine Tumor Society have attempted to improve the standardization of the classification, grading, and staging of NETs.[2–4]

Disclosures: The authors herewith certifies that have no non-financial or commercial, proprietary, or financial interest in the products or companies described in the manuscript. The authors did not receive grants or a consultant honorarium to conduct the study, write the manuscript or otherwise assist in the development of the manuscript.

[a] PET Unit, Department of Nuclear Medicine, Santa Maria della Misericordia Hospital, Viale Tre Martiri 140, Rovigo 45100, Italy; [b] Department of Nuclear Medicine, All India Institute of Medical Sciences, New Delhi 110029, India; [c] Department of Radiology, University of Pennsylvania, 3400 Spruce Street, Philadelphia, PA 19104, USA

* Corresponding author. Department of Nuclear Medicine, PET/CT Centre, Radiology, Neuroradiology, Medical Physics, Santa Maria della Misericordia Hospital, Viale Tre Martiri, 140, Rovigo 45100, Italy.
*E-mail address:* rubello.domenico@azisanrovigo.it

PET Clin 9 (2014) 1–9
http://dx.doi.org/10.1016/j.cpet.2013.08.010
1556-8598/14/$ – see front matter

Essentially, the new accepted classification consists of 3 main histologic categories: low-grade NETs (grade 1), intermediate-grade NETs (grade 2), and high-grade NETs (grade 3, also called *neuroendocrine carcinoma*). Grade 1 and 2 are considered well-differentiated tumors (previously defined as either carcinoid or atypical carcinoid), whereas grade 3 is considered poorly differentiated **(Table 1)**.[5,6]

Differentiation refers to the extent that the neoplastic cells look like their non-neoplastic counterparts; for example, well-differentiated NETs have characteristic organoid architecture, well-differentiated cytology, and produce abundant neurosecretory granules. Grading, conversely, refers to the biologic tumor's vigor; for example, high-grade tumors are extremely aggressive.

The proliferative rate expressed by mitotic count and Ki-67 index (see **Table 1**) has been repeatedly shown to provide significant prognostic information for NETs[7,8]; most systems of grading rely extensively on the proliferative rate to separate low-, intermediate-, and high-grade tumors.

The new WHO classification, published in 2010,[1] has introduced some new considerations about NETs. Firstly, the terms *benign* and *malignant* have been eliminated because neuroendocrine neoplasms are all potentially malignant. Therefore, all neuroendocrine neoplasms that were previously regarded as benign have now been considered in the incidence data (for example, Surveillance, Epidemiology, and End Results [SEER] data). Secondly, the term *atypical carcinoid* is not recommended and it cannot be used for G2 neuroendocrine tumors. Even though *endocrine* and *neuroendocrine* are essentially synonymous, the use of *neuroendocrine* has been once again recommended. The neoplasms composed of both neuroendocrine cells and nonendocrine components (usually adenocarcinoma structures) are classified as mixed adenoneuroendocrine carcinomas (note that neuroendocrine component should exceed at least 30% of all cells).

NETs could affect almost every apparatus through the body, but the most common ones arise from the duodenum, ileum, pancreas, bronchus, colon and rectum, stomach, thymus, and heart.

A particular subdivision of NETs is represented by functioning and nonfunctioning tumors. Non-functioning NETs may not present with clinical symptoms until they produce tumor mass effects at a late stage of growth. Functioning NETs (mostly pancreatic NETs) produce symptoms, sometimes remarkable, because of the excess release of various hormones and biologic amines by the tumor into the blood (histology specific, such as insulin, gastrin, vasoactive intestinal peptide, somatostatin, and glucagons, or generic, like serotonin, prostaglandin, and parathyroid hormone–releasing peptide).

Some functioning NETs could result from a background of multiple endocrine neoplasia (MEN); for example, duodenal gastrinoma could be associated with Zollinger-Ellison syndrome within MEN-1, and it is invariably multicentric, different from the sporadic type.[9]

## Epidemiology

The overall incidence rate of NETs has increased since 1975,[10,11] although it is uncertain if this tendency is caused by the advent of new diagnostic instrumentations, new NET definitions and classifications, the increased understanding among physicians, or an actual increase in NET incidence. The SEER database analysis shows an impressive 5-fold increase in the diagnosed incidence of NETs from 1973 to 2004,[12] and NETs' incidence is predicted to persist growing at a faster rate than other malignancies.[11] NETs are, of course, quite rare, accounting for only 0.5% of all malignancies[13]; but surprisingly, their prevalence is higher than gastric and pancreatic tumors combined.[14]

The greater part of NETs occurs in the gastrointestinal tract (about 67%, most of which are in the small intestine) and in the lungs (about 25%).[13] NETs of the rectum and appendix usually have a good prognosis, whereas NETs of the colon have

**Table 1**
**Differentiation and grading of NETs**

| Differentiation | Grade | Ki-67 Index[a] (%) | Mitotic Count (10 HPF)[b] (%) |
|---|---|---|---|
| Well differentiate | Low grade (G1) | ≤2 | <2 |
| | Intermediate grade (G2) | 3–20 | 2–20 |
| Poorly differentiate | High grade (G3) | >20 | >20 |

*Abbreviation:* HPF, high-power field.
[a] MIB1 antibody; percentage of 2000 tumor cells in areas of highest nuclear labeling.
[b] 10 HPF = 2 mm$^2$, at least 40 fields (at 40 × magnification) evaluated in areas of highest mitotic density.

the lowest life expectancy (67.4% of 5-year disease-specific survival).[10]

The prognosis is then obviously associated with the stage: 93% of 5-year survival in local disease, 74% in regional disease, and 19% in metastatic disease.[13]

## Markers

Biochemical NETs markers are substances secreted by the tumor that circulate in the blood and can be used for diagnosis and evaluation.

NETs markers can be an expression of nonfunctional NETs, like chromogranin A (CgA), neuron-specific enolase (NSE), 5-Hydroxyindoleacetic acid (5-HIAA), synaptophysin, neurokinin, pancreatic polypeptide, neurotensin, and $\alpha$ and $\beta$ human chorionic gonadotropin. Some of these proteins have shown a high accuracy in diagnosing NETs. Currently, CgA is the most accurate marker in diagnosis and for prognosis of NETs and it is suggested to be used for disease monitoring.[15] An article by Campana and coworkers[16] demonstrated that CgA could have a very high accuracy (sensitivity of 85% and specificity of 96%) using a proper cutoff (84–87 U/L) that helps to discriminate patients with elevated CgA as a result of other non-neoplastic disease (like chronic atrophic gastritis).[16] Among the other markers, 5-HIAA has a high specificity but low sensitivity (with the exception of ileal NETs); NSE shows its best sensitivity for poorly differentiated NETs.

In cases of carcinoid syndrome or specific syndrome of pancreatic NETs (**Table 2**), other markers are involved: gastrin, insulin, vasoactive intestinal peptide, and glucagon.[17]

## Radiopharmaceuticals and Protocols

Nuclear medicine plays a pivotal role in the imaging and treatment of NET. Considerable advances have been made in the imaging of NET with radiotracers, but to find the ideal imaging method with increased sensitivity and better topographic localization of the primary and metastatic disease remains the ultimate goal of research. The increasing understanding of the molecular basis of NET, especially the expression of somatostatin receptors (SSTR) in NET, fostered the development and introduction of a multitude of single-photon emission computed tomography (SPECT) and positron emission tomography (PET) tracers, which have significantly improved the ability for imaging these neoplastic lesions with high spatial resolution.

### SPECT radiotracers

Radioiodinated metaiodobenzylguanidine (MIBG) was the first radiopharmaceutical to be applied for imaging and therapy for some NET.[18] [123]I- and [131]I-MIBG have been used to image NET since the early 1980s. When it was first developed, MIBG was used to detect chromaffin cell tumors, such as pheochromocytomas and neuroblastomas.[19] In a review of 10 years of experience with MIBG scintigraphy, a median detection rate of 50% and sensitivity of 76% were reported for carcinoid tumors.[20] The mechanism of MIBG

---

**Table 2**
**NETs symptoms and syndromes**

|  | Clinical Features | Markers |
|---|---|---|
| Functioning NETs causing carcinoid syndromes | Diarrhea, flushing, wheezing, hypotension | Serotonin, histamine, prostaglandin, parathyroid hormone–releasing peptide |
| Bone metastasis | Pain, bone fracture | Bone alkaline phosphatase |
| Insulinoma | Hypoglycemia | Insulin |
| Gastrinoma (Zollinger-Ellison) | Diarrhea, abdominal pain (gastric ulcer) | Gastrin |
| VIPoma (Verner-Morrison) | Watery diarrhea, hypokalemia | Vasoactive intestinal polypeptide |
| Glucagonoma | Anemia, glucose intolerance, diabetes, weight loss | Glucagon |
| Somatostatinoma | Diabetes, diarrhea, steatorrhea, cholelithiasis | Somatostatin |
| GHRFoma | Acromegaly | Growth hormone–releasing factor |
| ACTHoma | Cushing syndrome | ACTH |

*Abbreviation:* ACTH, adrenocorticotropic hormone.

accumulation is a combination of uptake by the norepinephrine transporter and passive diffusion, with affinity for vesicular monoamine transporter incorporating MIBG into neurosecretory vesicles.[21] Typically, 370 MBq ([123]I-MIBG) or 37 to 74 MBq ([131]I-MIBG) of the radiopharmaceutical is administered by slow intravenous injection. Scanning is usually performed after 48 hours for [131]I-MIBG or after 24 hours for [123]I-MIBG, preferentially including SPECT imaging. [123]I-MIBG is better suited when compared with [131]I for gamma camera imaging. MIBG is especially suitable for imaging tumors with functional activity, such as pheochromocytomas, functioning paragangliomas, neuroblastomas, medullary thyroid carcinomas, and carcinoids. MIBG was found to have a limited role in NETs of the pancreas.[22] MIBG examinations are associated with practical constraints, such as long imaging times, thyroid blockage, and need for withdrawal of interfering medications. Also, MIBG in other NETs has been shown to have a lower sensitivity than the more frequently used [111]In somatostatin receptor scintigraphy (SRS).[23] Consequently, the main indication for MIBG imaging is in selecting lesions with high MIBG uptake for MIBG-targeted radionuclide therapy.

The first report of overexpression of SSTR on tumor tissue was published in 1984.[24] Six different SSTR have been identified (SSTR1, 2A, 2B, 3, 4, 5) in humans; a predominance of SSTR2 and/or SSTR1 was noted with Gastro-entero-pancreatic (GEP)-NET.[25] The first successful in vivo imaging of these NETs expressing SSTR with[123]I-[Tyr[3]] octreotide was published in 1989,[26] which led to the clinical utility for tumor localization using SRS.[27] However, relatively high nonreceptor-based uptake in the liver and intestinal uptake (both can obscure occult pathology) was an important drawback. Therefore, a radiolabeled somatostatin analogue with better characteristics, [111]In-diethylenetriamine pentaacetic acid (DTPA)-octreotide, was developed, which showed an improved biodistribution when compared with the initially used [123]I-Tyr3-octreotide, with a shift from a gastrointestinal excretion that interferes with tumor uptake in the abdominal region to a prevalent renal excretion. The cyclic octapeptide octreotide was the first Somatostatin analogue to be used in clinical practice. In 1994, [111]In-DTPA-octreotide (Octreoscan, Mallinckrodt, St Louis, MO) was approved by the Food and Drug Administration as an imaging agent for SSTR-positive NET.[28] Since then, [111]In-DTPA-octreotide was regarded as the gold standard in nuclear imaging for patients with GEP-NETs.[27] The somatostatin analogue octreotide binds with high affinity to SSTR2, which is essential for imaging tumors with SRS.[29] Over the last 3 decades, [111]In-octreotide scintigraphy has become a key imaging modality in staging and restaging NET. The recommended administered activity is 185 to 222 MBq in adults and 5 MBq/kg in children. Image acquisition is performed at 4 and 24 hours and up to 48 hours for more accurate imaging when significant bowl activity is present.

Although [111]In-DTPA-octreotide scintigraphy was successful, the acyclic bifunctional chelators DTPA conjugated via one of the carboxyl group with the targeting vector molecule turned out to be unsuitable with any other radio metals than [111]In because of its in vivo instability.[30] This situation led to the introduction of 1,4,7,10-tetraazacyclodecane-1,4,7,10-tetraacetic acid (DOTA), a universal chelator capable of forming stable complexes with radiotracers of the metal group, such as [111]In, [67]Ga, [68]Ga, [64]Cu, [90]Y, and [177]Lu,[31] which was a step forward in labeling peptides. [111]In–DOTA radiopharmaceuticals include [111]In-DOTA-octreotide ([111]In-DOTA-OC), [111]In-DOTA-1-Nal[3]-octreotide ([111]In-DOTA-NOC) and [111]In-DOTA-Tyr[3]-octreotide ([111]In-DOTA-TOC), which have varying profiles regarding SSTR subtype affinity and variable results. Subsequent research to improve the image resolution and availability identified alternative agents to [111]In-DTPA-octreotide scintigraphy leading to the development of [99m]Tc–labeled somatostatin analogues: [99m]Tc-hydrazinonicotinyl-Tyr[3]-octreotide ([99m]Tc-HYNIC-TOC), [99m]Tc-hydrazinonicotinyl-Tyr[3]-octreotate ([99m]Tc-HYNIC-TATE), and [99m]Tc-depreotide.[32–34] The most important advantages of the use of [99m]Tc include no expense of producing [111]In in a cyclotron and no need to wait 24 to 48 hours after injection for optimal detection of tumors. However, [99m]Tc-depreotide and [111]In-DOTA-lanreotide are not ideally suited for imaging abdominal NET primarily because of their diminished sensitivity compared with [111]In-DTPA-octreotide.[35,36]

SRS has a high sensitivity for detecting typical carcinoid and gastrointestinal pancreatic NET, particularly, gastrinomas, nonfunctioning NET, and functioning endocrine pancreatic tumors except insulinomas (because of the lack of SSTR2 expression).[37] Other peptides, like [111]Indium-minigastrin, targeting the pentagastrin-binding receptor (CCK2), or radiolabeled exendin-4, targeting the glucagonlike peptide 1 receptor, which displays a high sensitivity for insulinomas, have been proposed for peptide imaging.[38] In another recent study, gastrin-receptor scintigraphy provided additional information as compared with SSTR scintigraphy in selected patients with NET.[39] After the successful introduction of SRS in the diagnosis and staging of NET, the next logical step was to target the SSTR for therapy. Therefore, the first peptide receptor radionuclide therapy (PRRT) was performed with high administered activity of $^{111}$In-DTPA-octreotide.[40]

*Evolution of scanner for SPECT radiotracers*
Planar scintigraphy is one area of scintigraphic imaging whereby fusion with anatomic modalities has not penetrated to any significant degree. Traditionally, a 2-dimensional planar whole-body image is acquired followed by SPECT through regions of interest. The latter enables 3-dimensional reconstruction and improved tumor to background contrast. Modern SPECT imaging with $^{111}$In yields sensitivities in excess of 80% for carcinoid tumor metastases.[41] A recent development is the introduction of improved hybrid modality, SPECT/computed tomography (CT), which has the advantages of better sensitivity and specificity. The main advantages of SPECT/CT are represented by better attenuation correction, increased specificity, and accurate depiction of the localization of disease and of possible involvement of adjacent tissues. Superior diagnostic accuracy of SPECT/CT over planar and SPECT imaging has been consistently reported, thereby improving diagnostic confidence and reporter agreement impacting patient-management decisions.[42–45] These advantages are especially true for pancreatic and lymph node lesions. Specificity is also increased by confirming physiologic localization to sites, such as bowel. SSTR analogues and MIBG remain front-line SPECT radiotracers in the imaging of enterochromaffin and chromaffin NET, respectively; their utility has been further augmented in recent years by the increasing availability of SPECT/CT technology.

*PET radiotracers*
Although SRS showed a higher accuracy than CT[27] for NET diagnosis, the development of novel PET tracers specific for NET has revolutionized the diagnostic approach. In the past decade, several beta-emitting tracers have been developed for NET imaging, mainly as a consequence of the marginal role of $^{18}$F-fluorodeoxyglucose ($^{18}$F-FDG) for the assessment of these tumors secondary to $^{18}$F-FDG's low sensitivity for detecting tumors with slow growth and malignant potential.[46] Among these radiopharmaceuticals, gallium-68-labeled somatostatin analogues are increasingly used. Research and interest in $^{68}$Ge and $^{68}$Ga started in the early 1950s.[47,48] In 1960, the $^{68}$Ge/$^{68}$Ga generator was first described[49]; a revival started in the 1970s, when several other $^{68}$Ge/$^{68}$Ga generator systems were developed.[50] The availability of PET radiolabeled pharmaceuticals by the introduction of $^{68}$Ga in radiopharmacy, independent of an on-site cyclotron, opened new applications and possibilities. The earliest NET $^{68}$Ga-DOTATOC PET studies were conducted by Hoffman and colleagues,[51] showing high tumor-to-nontumor ratios and identifying metastatic lesions not uncovered by SPECT or conventional imaging. First introduced in clinical application in 2005, $^{68}$Ga-DOTATOC was reported to present a high tumor-to-nontumor contrast and a higher sensitivity compared with SRS.[51,52] Other $^{68}$Ga somatostatin analogues were developed to increase their sensitivity, including $^{68}$Ga-DOTATATE and $^{68}$Ga-DOTANOC.[53,54] $^{68}$Ga-DOTANOC has revealed promising results in preliminary studies for the main clinical indications: staging NET, suspected NET of unknown primary, follow-up, restaging, and finally for the pretreatment and posttreatment evaluation of receptor radionuclide therapies. PET/CT acquisition starts at 45 to 60 minutes after the intravenous injection of 100 to 200 MBq of the radiolabeled peptide. Somatostatin analogue therapy should be stopped before PET/CT: short-acting analogues for 3 days before PET/CT and long-acting analogues for 4 to 6 weeks. Another attractive radionuclide for PET imaging is $^{64}$Cu (physical half-life 12.7 hours), which can be obtained by either a reactor or a medical cyclotron. Because of the high rate of lesion detection, sensitivity, and favorable dosimetry and pharmacokinetics, $^{64}$Cu-TETA-octreotide and $^{64}$Cu-DOTATOC have shown potential for PET imaging in patients with NET, which needs to be evaluated further.[55,56]

PET has several advantages over imaging methods that use gamma-emitting radiopharmaceuticals, such as $^{111}$In-pentetreotide or $^{123}$I-MIBG, including excellent signal-to-noise ratios, spatial resolution, and image quality. Also, good sensitivity of $^{68}$Ga-DOTANOC was reported especially for cases with an unusual anatomic localization[57] and small lesions, particularly at the node and bone level.[58] Other advantages include easy accessibility and availability of the $^{68}$Ga generator, a relatively short scanning time, and a relatively low radiation exposure.[59] It also provides relevant information of SSTR expression, which has a direct therapeutic implication with PRRT. Regarding potential pitfalls in image interpretation, it is important to notice that the presence of inflammation, reactive nodes, osteoblasts, benign meningiomas, accessory spleen, pancreatic uncinate process activity,[60] and physiologic activity at the adrenal level can cause false-positive results.

6-L-$^{18}$F-fluorodihydroxyphenylalanine ($^{18}$F-FDOPA), first introduced for imaging the striatonigral pathway in Parkinson disease, has been successfully used for PET imaging of NET. $^{18}$F-DOPA is concentrated by neuroendocrine tumors through a large neutral amino acid transporter (L-type amino acid transporter 1)[61] that is upregulated and highly active in the cells of these tumors. In 2001, Hoegerle and colleagues[62] reported that $^{18}$F-FDOPA PET allowed the detection of a higher number of gastrointestinal NET lesions as compared with SRS and $^{18}$F-FDG PET. False positives are rare with $^{18}$F-FDOPA PET, implicating higher tumor specificity than the somatostatin analogues or FDG, which are taken up by leucocytes in inflammatory lesions. $^{18}$F-FDOPA has demonstrated impressive results in differentiating between focal and diffuse disease in hyperinsulinism.[63] Generally, $^{18}$F-FDOPA PET is most sensitive in patients with functioning carcinoid tumors, chromaffin NET, medullary thyroid carcinoma (MTC) with calcitonin greater than 150 ng/mL,[64] and NET originating from the midgut.[62,65,66] It has a lower sensitivity for noncarcinoid NET, such as pancreatic islet cell tumors.[67] Difficulties in the requirement of modest radiochemistry expertise and high costs of FDOPA production limit its routine use. However, recently, the curie level of FDOPA production was achieved,[68] which needs to be experimented in routine practice. Another relative limitation of $^{18}$F-FDOPA PET/CT is that it is an imaging biomarker that does not offer a target for radionuclide-based therapies compared with peptide-labeled molecular imaging. Other PET radiotracers in this family include $^{11}$C-5-hydroxy- L-tryptophan ($^{11}$C-HTP), $^{11}$C-hydroxyephedrine ($^{11}$C-HED), $^{11}$C-epinephrine, and $^{18}$F-fluorodopamine ($^{18}$F-DA); but the shorter half-life of $^{11}$C and more complex radiosynthetic process for these radiotracers restricts their use to research applications.[21]

Because SSTR imaging does not only offer diagnostic information but can also be decisive for further treatment management, such as PRRT, in patients with GEP-NET, SSTR-PET is used as the initial functional imaging method. However, in patients with NET with negative SSTR imaging, FDOPA-PET is considered a valuable second-line alternative.

Most poorly differentiated NETs are locally advanced or metastatic at presentation and exhibit aggressive histologic features. Because they express somatostatin receptors less frequently, SRS and SSRT PET is usually negative, whereas $^{18}$F-FDG PET seems to be the best method of evaluating disease spread and guiding further treatment. Study is acquired after an uptake time of 60 minutes following intravenous injection of 370 Mbq of $^{18}$F-FDG in 6-hour fastened patients. The $^{18}$F-FDG PET semiquantitative parameter standardized uptake value has been demonstrated to be an independent predictive factor for progression-free survival.[69] In fact, $^{18}$F-FDG PET, providing valuable prognostic information, may select patients with more aggressive disease that need to be treated with chemotherapy. In this scenario, having a negative FDG image is great news for patients with NET because this means that the tumor is highly differentiated and, therefore, has a better prognosis. Such as for other cancers, it has to be emphasized that a negative FDG scan in this particular population is a true negative result and not a false-negative finding.[70] Another clinical setting in which $^{18}$F-FDG PET may be useful is for the detection of atypical lung carcinoids,[71] aggressive MTC with short calcitonin doubling times, or with various degrees of somatostatin receptor expression, poorly differentiated NET, and endocrine small cell or oat cell tumors of the thymus[72] and prostate.[73]

Recently, new knowledge on cancer biology has been raised: tumors can be composed of different subpopulations of cells with different degrees of differentiation, growth rates, and response to treatments. There could be both an *intertumor* heterogeneity (for example, different biologic behaviors between various lesions of the same malignancy) and an *intratumor* heterogeneity, which has been relatively less well investigated probably because of the lack of available ad hoc techniques in the past decades. Molecular imaging is based on in vivo tracking of various metabolic pathways (such as glycolysis, receptorial affinity, proliferation rate, cells membrane formation, fatty acid metabolism, and so forth) through different and specific radiopharmaceuticals; therefore, it is the ideal instrumentation for investigating the heterogeneity of cancer tissue. For example, it can happen that in the same patient some lesions are well visualized by somatostatin-analogue compounds, others by dopaminergic agents, and finally those that are undifferentiated are highlighted by FDG. These observations bring many implications not only on the choice of the right diagnostic methods but, above all, for selecting and tailoring various treatment options.[74]

### Evolution of scanner for PET radiotracers

The main disadvantage of SPECT is probably the still low resolution of the image, which is prone to artifacts and attenuation, limiting the ability to detect tiny lesions. SPECT also does not provide a quantifiable estimate of tumor metabolism and tracer uptake. Thus, PET has been growing rapidly in the imaging of NET, paralleled by great efforts toward the development of new tracers. After the successful introduction of in-line hybrid PET/CT scanners, investigators extended the concept of dedicated hybrid imaging systems to SPECT/CT and, more recently, PET/magnetic resonance (MR) imaging systems. PET/CT is the superior methodology for staging and detection of primary tumors of undetermined location. SPECT and SPECT/CT imaging with [111]In-pentetreotide or [123]I-MIBG will likely be replaced in the future by PET/CT with [68]Ga-labeled octreopeptides and [18]F-FDOPA, as hypothesized by Alavi and colleagues in 2008.[75] PET/CT and PET/MR imaging using the positron emitter [124]I-MIBG[76,77] in NET evaluation has been reported. Recently, simultaneous [68]Ga-DOTATOC PET/MR imaging acquisition was shown to have special advantages in the characterization of abdominal lesions.[78] Thus, hybrid imaging, such as PET/CT or PET/MR imaging, will play an important role in the future.

## REFERENCES

1. Bosman F, Carneiro F, Hruban R, et al, editors. WHO classification of tumours of the digestive system. Lyon (France): IARC Press; 2010.
2. Sobin L, Gospodarowicz M, Wittekind C. TNM classification of malignant tumours. 7th edition. Bognor Regis (United Kingdom): Wiley-Blackwell; 2009.
3. Edge SB, Byrd DR, Compton CC, et al. AJCC cancer staging manual. New York: Springer; 2010.
4. Salazar R, Wiedenmann B, Rindi G, et al. ENETS 2011 consensus guidelines for the management of patients with digestive neuroendocrine tumors: an update. Neuroendocrinology 2012;95:71–3.
5. Rindi G, Klöppel G, Ahlman H, et al. TNM staging of foregut (neuro) endocrine tumors: a consensus proposal including a grading system. Virchows Arch 2006;449:395–401.
6. Klimstra DS, Modlin IR, Coppola D, et al. The pathologic classification of neuroendocrine tumors: a review of nomenclature, grading, and staging systems. Pancreas 2010;39:707–12.
7. Pape UF, Berndt U, Muller-Nordhorn J, et al. Prognostic factors of long-term outcome in gastroenteropancreatic neuroendocrine tumours. Endocr Relat Cancer 2008;15:1083–97.
8. Ferrone CR, Tang LH, Tomlinson J, et al. Determining prognosis in patients with pancreatic endocrine neoplasms: can the WHO classification system be simplified? J Clin Oncol 2007;25:5609–15.
9. Pipeleers-Marichal M, Somers G, Willems G, et al. Gastrinomas in the duodenums of patients with multiple endocrine neoplasia type 1 and the Zollinger-Ellison syndrome. N Engl J Med 1990;322:723–7.
10. Tsikitis VL, Wertheim BC, Guerrero MA. Trends of incidence and survival of gastrointestinal neuroendocrine tumors in the United States: a SEER analysis. J Cancer 2012;3:292–302.
11. Modlin IM, Lye KD, Kidd M. A 5-decade analysis of 13,715 carcinoid tumors. Cancer 2003;97:934–59.
12. Yao JC, Hassan M, Phan A, et al. One hundred years after "carcinoid": epidemiology of and prognostic factors for neuroendocrine tumors in 35,825 cases in the United States. J Clin Oncol 2008;26:3063–72.
13. Taal BG, Visser O. Epidemiology of neuroendocrine tumours. Neuroendocrinology 2004;80(Suppl 1):3–7.
14. National Cancer Institute, Surveillance, Epidemiology and End Results (SEER) stat fact sheets. Available at: www.seer.cancer.gov. Accessed January 17, 2012.
15. Ferolla P, Faggiano A, Mansueto G, et al. The biological characterization of neuroendocrine tumors: the role of neuroendocrine markers. J Endocrinol Invest 2008;31:277–86.
16. Campana D, Nori F, Piscitelli L, et al. Chromogranin A: is it a useful marker of neuroendocrine tumors? J Clin Oncol 2007;25:1967–73.
17. Shulkin BL, Thompson NW, Shapiro B, et al. Pheochromocytomas: imaging with 2-[fluorine-18]fluoro-2-deoxy-D-glucose PET. Radiology 1999;212:35–41.
18. Wieland DM, Wu JL, Brown LE, et al. Radiolabeled adrenergic neuron blocking agents: adrenomedullary imaging with 131I-iodobenzylguanidine. J Nucl Med 1980;21:349–53.
19. Hoefnagel CA, den Hartog Jager FC, Taal BG, et al. The role of I-131-MIBG in the diagnosis and therapy of carcinoids. Eur J Nucl Med 1987;13:187–91.
20. Modlin IM, Latich I, Zikusoka M, et al. Gastrointestinal carcinoids: the evolution of diagnostic strategies. J Clin Gastroenterol 2006;40:572–82.
21. Koopmans KP, Neels ON, Kema IP, et al. Molecular imaging in neuroendocrine tumors: molecular uptake mechanisms and clinical results. Crit Rev Oncol Hematol 2009;71:199–213.
22. Kaltsas G, Korbonits M, Heintz E, et al. Comparison of somatostatin analog and metaiodobenzylguanidine radionuclides in the diagnosis and localization of advanced neuroendocrine tumors. J Clin Endocrinol Metab 2001;86:895–902.
23. Modlin IM, Kidd M, Latich I, et al. Current status of gastrointestinal carcinoids. Gastroenterology 2005;128:1717–51.
24. Reubi JC, Landolt AM. High density of somatostatin receptors in pituitary tumors from acromegalic patients. J Clin Endocrinol Metab 1984;59:1148–51.
25. Reubi JC, Waser B, Schaer JC, et al. Somatostatin receptor sst1-sst5 expression in normal and

neoplastic human tissues using receptor autoradiography with subtype-selective ligands. Eur J Nucl Med 2001;28:836–46.

26. Krenning EP, Bakker WH, Breeman WA, et al. Localisation of endocrine-related tumours with radioiodinated analogue of somatostatin. Lancet 1989;1:242–4.

27. Krenning EP, Kwekkeboom DJ, Bakker WH, et al. Somatostatin receptor scintigraphy with [111In-DTPA-D-Phe1]- and [123I-Tyr3]-octreotide: the Rotterdam experience with more than 1000 patients. Eur J Nucl Med 1993;20:716–31.

28. Rufini V, Calcagni ML, Baum RP. Imaging of neuroendocrine tumors. Semin Nucl Med 2006; 36:228–47.

29. Hofland LJ, Lamberts SW, van Hagen PM, et al. Crucial role for somatostatin receptor subtype 2 in determining the uptake of [111In-DTPA-D-Phe1] octreotide in somatostatin receptor-positive organs. J Nucl Med 2003;44:1315–21.

30. Harrison A, Walker CA, Parker D, et al. The in vivo release of 90Y from cyclic and acyclic ligand-antibody conjugates. Int J Rad Appl Instrum B 1991;18:469–76.

31. Wild D, Schmitt JS, Ginj M, et al. DOTA-NOC, a high-affinity ligand of somatostatin receptor subtypes 2, 3 and 5 for labelling with various radiometals. Eur J Nucl Med Mol Imaging 2003;30(10): 1338–47.

32. Hubalewska-Dydejczyk A, Fröss-Baron K, Mikołajczak R, et al. 99mTc-EDDA/HYNIC-octreotate scintigraphy, an efficient method for the detection and staging of carcinoid tumours: results of 3 years' experience. Eur J Nucl Med Mol Imaging 2006;33:1123–33.

33. Gabriel M, Hausler F, Bale R, et al. Image fusion analysis of (99m)Tc-HYNIC-Tyr(3)-octreotide SPECT and diagnostic CT using an immobilisation device with external markers in patients with endocrine tumours. Eur J Nucl Med Mol Imaging 2005; 32:1440–51.

34. Lebtahi R, Le Cloirec J, Houzard C, et al. Detection of neuroendocrine tumors: 99mTc-P829 scintigraphy compared with 111In-pentetreotide scintigraphy. J Nucl Med 2002;43:889–95.

35. Kwekkeboom DJ, Kam BL, van Essen M, et al. Somatostatin-receptor-based imaging and therapy of gastroenteropancreatic neuroendocrine tumors. Endocr Relat Cancer 2010;17:R53–73.

36. Menda Y, Kahn D. Somatostatin receptor imaging of non-small cell lung cancer with 99mTc depreotide. Semin Nucl Med 2002;32:92–6.

37. Lebtahi R, Cadiot G, Sarda L, et al. Clinical impact of somatostatin receptor scintigraphy in the management of patients with neuroendocrine gastroenteropancreatic tumors. J Nucl Med 1997;38: 853–8.

38. Reubi JC, Maecke HR. Peptide-based probes for cancer imaging. J Nucl Med 2008;49:1735–8.

39. Gotthardt M, Behe MP, Grass J, et al. Added value of gastrin receptor scintigraphy in comparison to somatostatin receptor scintigraphy in patients with carcinoids and other neuroendocrine tumours. Endocr Relat Cancer 2006;13:1203–11.

40. Krenning EP, Kooij PP, Bakker WH, et al. Radiotherapy with a radiolabeled somatostatin analogue, [111In-DTPA-D-Phe1]-octreotide. A case history. Ann N Y Acad Sci 1994;733:496–506.

41. Kaltsas G, Rockall A, Papadogias D, et al. Recent advances in radiological and radionuclide imaging and therapy of neuroendocrine tumours. Eur J Endocrinol 2004;151:15–27.

42. Ingui CJ, Shah NP, Oates ME. Endocrine neoplasm scintigraphy: added value of fusing SPECT/CT images compared with traditional side-by-side analysis. Clin Nucl Med 2006;31:665–72.

43. Patel CN, Chowdhury FU, Scarsbrook AF. Clinical utility of hybrid SPECT-CT in endocrine neoplasia. AJR Am J Roentgenol 2008;190:815–24.

44. Apostolova I, Riethdorf S, Buchert R, et al. SPECT/CT stabilizes the interpretation of somatostatin receptor scintigraphy findings: a retrospective analysis of inter-rater agreement. Ann Nucl Med 2010;24:477–83.

45. Castaldi P, Rufini V, Treglia G, et al. Impact of 111In-DTPA-octreotide SPECT/CT fusion images in the management of neuroendocrine tumours. Radiol Med 2008;113:1056–67.

46. Adams S, Baum R, Rink T, et al. Limited value of fluorine-18 fluorodeoxyglucose positron emission tomography for the imaging of neuroendocrine tumors. Eur J Nucl Med 1998;25:79–83.

47. Rosenfeld G. Studies of the metabolism of germanium. Arch Biochem Biophys 1954;48:84–94.

48. Roesch F, Riss PJ. The renaissance of the Ge/Ga radionuclide generator initiates new developments in Ga radiopharmaceutical chemistry. Curr Top Med Chem 2010;10:1633–68.

49. Gleason GI. A positron cow. Int J Appl Radiat Isot 1960;8:90–4.

50. Fani M, Andre JP, Maecke HR. 68Ga-PET: a powerful generator-based alternative to cyclotron-based PET radiopharmaceuticals. Contrast Media Mol Imaging 2008;3:67–77.

51. Hofmann M, Maecke H, Borner R, et al. Biokinetics and imaging with the somatostatin receptor PET radioligand (68)Ga-DOTATOC: preliminary data. Eur J Nucl Med 2001;28:1751–7.

52. Kowalski J, Henze M, Schuhmacher J, et al. Evaluation of positron emission tomography imaging using [68Ga]-DOTA-D Phe (1)-Tyr (3)-Octreotide in comparison to [111In]-DTPAOC SPECT, First results in patients with neuroendocrine tumors. Mol Imaging Biol 2003;5:42–8.

53. Bushnell DL, Baum RP. Standard imaging techniques for neuroendocrine tumors. Endocrinol Metab Clin North Am 2011;40:153–62.
54. Wild D, Mäcke HR, Waser B, et al. 68Ga-DOTA-NOC: a first compound for PET imaging with high affinity for somatostatin receptor subtypes 2 and 5. Eur J Nucl Med Mol Imaging 2005;32:724.
55. Anderson CJ, Dehdashti F, Cutler PD, et al. 64Cu-TETA-octreotide as a PET imaging agent for patients with neuroendocrine tumors. J Nucl Med 2001;42:213–21.
56. Hanaoka H, Tominaga H, Yamada K, et al. Evaluation of (64)Cu-labeled DOTA-D-Phe(1)-Tyr (3)-octreotide ((64)Cu-DOTA-TOC) for imaging somatostatin receptor-expressing tumors. Ann Nucl Med 2009;23:559–67.
57. Fanti S, Ambrosini V, Tomassetti P, et al. Evaluation of unusual neuroendocrine tumours by means of [68Ga]DOTA-NOC PET. Biomed Pharmacother 2008;62:667–71.
58. Ambrosini V, Tomassetti P, Castellucci P, et al. Comparison between [68Ga]DOTA-NOC and [18F] DOPA PET for the detection of gastro-enteropancreatic and lung neuro-endocrine tumours. Eur J Nucl Med Mol Imaging 2008;35:1431–8.
59. Krausz Y, Freedman N, Rubinstein R, et al. 68Ga-DOTA-NOC PET/CT imaging of neuroendocrine tumors: comparison with 111In-DTPA-octreotide (OctreoScan®). Mol Imaging Biol 2011;13:583–93.
60. Hofman MS, Kong G, Neels OC, et al. High management impact of Ga-68 DOTATATE (GaTate) PET/CT for imaging neuroendocrine and other somatostatin expressing tumours. J Med Imaging Radiat Oncol 2012;56:40–7.
61. Jager PL, Chirakal R, Marriott CJ, et al. 6-L-18F-fluorodihydroxyphenylalanine PET in neuroendocrine tumors: basic aspects and emerging clinical applications. J Nucl Med 2008;49:573–86.
62. Hoegerle S, Altehoefer C, Ghanem N, et al. Whole-body 18F dopa PET for detection of gastrointestinal carcinoid tumors. Radiology 2001;220:373–80.
63. Mohnike W, Barthlen W, Mohnike K, et al. Positron emission tomography/computed tomography diagnostics by means of fluorine-18-L-dihydroxyphenylalanine in congenital hyperinsulinism. Semin Pediatr Surg 2011;20:23–7.
64. American Thyroid Association Guidelines Task Force, Kloos RT, Eng C, Evans DB, et al. Medullary thyroid cancer: management guidelines of the American Thyroid Association. Thyroid 2009;19:565–612.
65. Montravers F, Grahek D, Kerrou K, et al. Can fluorodihydroxyphenylalanine PET replace somatostatin receptor scintigraphy in patients with digestive endocrine tumors? J Nucl Med 2006;47:1455–62.
66. Koopmans KP, Neels OC, Kema IP, et al. Improved staging of patients with carcinoid and islet cell tumors with 18F-dihydroxy-phenyl-alanine and 11C-5-hydroxy-tryptophan positron emission tomography. J Clin Oncol 2008;26:1489–95.
67. Balogova S, Talbot JN, Nataf V, et al. (18)F-fluorodihydroxyphenylalanine vs other radiopharmaceuticals for imaging neuroendocrine tumours according to their type. Eur J Nucl Med Mol Imaging 2013;40:943–66.
68. Libert LC, Franci X, Plenevaux AR, et al. Production at the Curie level of no-carrier-added 6-18F-fluoro-L-dopa. J Nucl Med 2013;54(7):1154–61.
69. Garin E, Le Jeune F, Devillers A, et al. Predictive value of 18F-FDG PET and somatostatin receptor scintigraphy in patients with metastatic endocrine tumors. J Nucl Med 2009;50:858–64.
70. Kwee TC, Basu S, Saboury B, et al. A new dimension of FDG-PET interpretation: assessment of tumor biology. Eur J Nucl Med Mol Imaging 2011;38(6):1158–70.
71. Kayani I, Conry BG, Groves AM, et al. A comparison of 68Ga-DOTATATE and 18F-FDG PET/CT in pulmonary neuroendocrine tumors. J Nucl Med 2009;50:1927–32.
72. Fujishita T, Kishida M, Taki H, et al. Detection of primary and metastatic lesions by [18F]fluoro-2-deoxy-D-glucose PET in a patient with thymic carcinoid. Respirology 2007;12:928–30.
73. de Carvalho Flamini R, Yamaga L, Mello ME, et al. F-18 FDG PET/CT imaging in small cell prostate cancer. Clin Nucl Med 2010;35:452–3.
74. Basu S, Kwee TC, Gatenby R, et al. Evolving role of molecular imaging with PET in detecting and characterizing heterogeneity of cancer tissue at the primary and metastatic sites, a plausible explanation for failed attempts to cure malignant disorders. Eur J Nucl Med Mol Imaging 2011;38(6):987–91.
75. Alavi A, Basu S. Planar and SPECT imaging in the era of PET and PET-CT: can it survive the test of time? Eur J Nucl Med Mol Imaging 2008;35(8):1554–9.
76. Lee CL, Wahnishe H, Sayre GA, et al. Radiation dose estimation using preclinical imaging with 124I-metaiodobenzylguanidine (MIBG) PET. Med Phys 2010;37:4861–7.
77. Hartung-Knemeyer V, Rosenbaum-Krumme S, Buchbender C, et al. Malignant pheochromocytoma imaging with [124I]mIBG PET/MR. J Clin Endocrinol Metab 2012;97:3833–4.
78. Beiderwellen KJ, Poeppel TD, Hartung-Knemeyer V, et al. Simultaneous 68Ga-DOTATOC PET/MRI in patients with gastroenteropancreatic neuroendocrine tumors: initial results. Invest Radiol 2013;48:273–9.

# Single-Photon Emission Computed Tomography Tracers in the Diagnostics of Neuroendocrine Tumors

Giovanna Pepe, MD[a], Emilio Bombardieri, MD[b],
Alice Lorenzoni, MD[b], Arturo Chiti, MD[a],*

KEYWORDS

- mIBG • Somatostatin • Somatostatin analogues • Pentetreotide

KEY POINTS

- Neuroendocrine tumors constitute a multisided, complex world, which has long been challenging for physicians.
- Different imaging strategies have been developed targeting the unique features of this group of rare diseases.
- Efforts have been made to study metabolic characteristics and receptor expression on the tumor surface, with knowledge still growing as a result of the implementation of fusion imaging and development of more detailed positron emission tomography tracers for NETs.
- In many countries, the scintigraphic study of NETs is still the most diffused and convenient technique to evaluate patients.

## INTRODUCTION

Under the term neuroendocrine tumors (NETs), several types of epithelial neoplasms with predominant neuroendocrine differentiation are grouped. These almost uncommon tumors, however heterogeneous, share their origin from neuroendocrine cells from the neural crest. On one hand, this is the reason why NETs can arise from different anatomic regions and tissues, given the broad distribution in the body of the neuroendocrine-derived cells. Thus, the common origin, because these tumors are part of the amine precursor and decarboxylation system (APUD), is why they produce hormones, despite their localization. As a consequence of this characteristic, different hormonal syndromes causing nonspecific symptoms may feature in the clinical presentation of these neoplasias.[1,2]

More often characterized by slow growing patterns and well-differentiated histologic features that correlate with a better prognosis, these tumors can also present with a range of poorly differentiated and more aggressive diseases.[3]

The incidence of this group of tumors accounts for about 5/100,000 cases, although it seems to have increased in the last 3 decades,[4] probably as a result of a greater awareness and new emphasis on its diagnostic-related issues.

The diagnosis of NETs has always been challenging, because of the wide range of clinical presentations and demonstrating the lesions

Conflict of Interest Statement: The authors have no conflict of interest to declare.
[a] Nuclear Medicine Department, Humanitas Clinical and Research Institute, Via A. Manzoni 56, 20089 Rozzano, Milan, Italy; [b] Nuclear Medicine Department, National Cancer Institute, Via G. venezian 1, Milan 20133, Italy
* Corresponding author. Humanitas Clinical and Research Institute, Via A. Manzoni 56, 20089 Rozzano, Milan, Italy.
*E-mail address:* arturo.chiti@humanitas.it

PET Clin 9 (2014) 11–26
http://dx.doi.org/10.1016/j.cpet.2013.08.011

has always been problematic mainly because of their small size, low rate of metabolism. and variable anatomic distribution. Conventional imaging sometimes shows results of nonunivocal interpretation.

However, functional imaging of NETs has become possible as a result of 2 fields of interest: the APUD metabolic features of the neuroendocrine cells and the discovery that most human NETs overexpress somatostatin (SS) receptors,[5] leading to the development of receptor-based imaging of NETs.

In this scenario, the contribution of nuclear medicine is essential for the in vivo detection of NETs.

The development of adrenomedullary radiopharmaceuticals took place mostly in the United States, in particular, at the University of Michigan; in Europe, most effort was given to the development and radiolabeling of SS analogues.

In this article, the origin and evolution of single-photon emission radiopharmaceuticals and diagnostic tools for the study of NETs are discussed.

## THE RADIOPHARMACEUTICALS
### A Metabolic Probe for the Study of NETs: Meta-[131]I-Benzylguanidine

The first synthesis of aralkylguanidines with an antiadrenergic effect dates back to 1967,[6] but it was between the end of the 1970s and the early 1980s that the successful radioiodination of these amines led to the first scintigraphic visualization of the adrenals in dogs[7] and later to the first imaging results in humans.[8,9]

The radiopharmaceutical used was meta-[131]I-benzylguanidine ([131]ImIBG), which derives from the combination of the benzyl group of bretylium and the guanidine group of guanethidine.

mIBG is an analogue of norepinephrine, sharing with this adrenergic hormone some characteristics of its molecular structure and the ability to enter the same metabolic pathway.

Norepinephrine is synthesized by normal adrenergic cells and stored in intracellular granules. Excretion follows an exocytosis mechanism. Reuptake is also possible via the vesicular monoamine transporters ($VMAT_1$ and $VMAT_2$).

Radiolabeled mIBG is taken up by VMAT and then stored in the secretory granules of the neuroendocrine cells[10] without being further metabolized significantly. The result is a specific concentration in these cells, which allows their visualization in contrast to nonadrenergic tissues.

Moreover, mIBG does not show relevant binding activity for postsynaptic receptors, hence the absence of a pharmacologic response.[11]

Both isotopes of iodine ([123]I and [131]I) commonly available in nuclear medicine diagnostic imaging are used for radiolabeling mIBG.

### SS and Its Analogues

SS, first described by Brazeau and colleagues,[12] is a cyclic hormone, a peptide naturally occurring in 2 forms (either 14 or 28 amino acids) in humans, with a short half-life of about 2 minutes. Its synthetic analogues, the octapeptides, octreotide and lanreotide, have a longer half-life (about 2 hours) and, therefore, have been developed for clinical use for both diagnostic and therapeutic purposes.[13,14]

SS and its analogues bind some specific receptors that belong to a family of G-protein coupled receptors; 5 subtypes have been identified: sstr1, sstr2, sstr3, sstr4, and sstr5[15]; their selective affinity toward native peptide and synthetic analogues is shown in **Table 1**.

Several studies have assessed the expression of these receptors on the tumor surface, and the results suggest that sstr2 is mostly represented on the surface of NETs, whereas ssrt3 is more widely diffused in human tumors.[16,17]

The possibility of radiolabeling the SS analogues enabled the in vivo investigation of the SS receptor distribution and, therefore, the imaging of NETs.

### Nuclear Medicine Receptor Imaging: an Outline

Toward the end of the 1980s, Krenning and the Rotterdam group[18] were the first to describe NETs in humans using scintigraphic planar images obtained with [123]I-Tyr3-octreotide, a radioiodinated SS analogue with a TYR substitution.[19,20] However, this tracer showed some weak points: high biliary excretion, leading to an accumulation in the bowel, making interpretation of the images more difficult; the high costs of [123]I production;

**Table 1**
**sstr subtype selectivity to endogenous SS and SS analogues**

| Agonist | Ki (nM) | | | | |
|---|---|---|---|---|---|
| | sstr1 | sstr2 | sstr3 | sstr4 | sstr5 |
| SS-14 | 1.1 | 1.3 | 1.6 | 0.53 | 0.9 |
| SS-28 | 2.2 | 4.1 | 6.1 | 1.1 | 0.07 |
| Octreotide | >1000 | 0.6 | 34.5 | >1000 | 7 |
| Lanreotide | >1000 | 0.8 | 107 | >1000 | 5.2 |
| Vapreotide | >1000 | 5.4 | 31 | 45 | 0.7 |
| Pasireotide (SOM-230) | 9.3 | 1.0 | 1.5 | >100 | 0.2 |

and the technically demanding labeling procedure. For this reason, other radiopharmaceuticals were developed.

The first tracer to be commercially available and registered in Europe for SS receptor imaging was [111]In-DTPA-D-Phe1-octreotide, also named [111]In-pentetreotide (OctreoScan, Mallinckrodt Medical, St. Louis, MO).

[111]In-Pentetreotide has a high affinity for sstr2 and lower affinity for sstr3, sstr5, and sstr4, respectively and shows high accuracy in the diagnosis and localization of primary NETs and secondary lesions.[21,22] In the United States, the Vanderbilt group in 1995[23] first reported the effectiveness of [111]In-pentetreotide as an imaging agent in carcinoids (a variety of NETs).

The clearance of [111]In-pentetreotide is mainly via the kidneys, and, therefore, there is less localization in the bowel, which makes interpretation of the images easier compared with [123]I-Tyr3-octreotide.[24]

However, [111]In does not represent an ideal isotope for imaging, especially because of its physical properties and, as a natural consequence of the widespread use of technetium 99m ([99m]Tc) in routine clinical practice, new tracers labeled with this isotope were developed.[25]

[99m]Tc-Depreotide, first named P829 and then registered (NeoTect, Bayer AG, Leverkusen, Germany; NeoSpect, Nycomed Pharma, Vienna, Austria) in both the United States and Europe for the characterization of lung solitary nodes, showed in a pilot study a sensitivity of 93% and a specificity of 89%.[26] Even despite its accuracy, this radiopharmaceutical was less effective compared with [111]In-pentetreotide, as reported by Lebtahi and colleagues.[27]

Other interesting scintigraphic results have been reported for [99m]Tc-EDDA/HYNIC-Tyr3-octreotide ([99m]Tc-EDDA/HYNIC-TOC) available in some European countries and registered in Poland (Tektrotyd, Polatom, Otwock, Poland) and for [99m]Tc-EDDA/HYNIC-Tyr3-octreotate ([99m]Tc-EDDA/HYNIC-TATE). These 2 tracers were compared by Cwikla and colleagues[28] and showed satisfactory results in a series of 12 patients, providing high-quality images, although [99m]Tc-EDDA/HYNIC-TATE seemed to be superior for nodal involvement and liver metastasis as a result of its lower lipophilicity.

[99m]Tc-EDDA/HYNIC-TOC was shown to be superior to [111]In-pentetreotide in a series of 75 patients.[29]

Generally, [99m]Tc-conjugate peptides seem to have several advantages compared with [111]In-pentetreotide, but the wide distribution of the latter has ensured its success as an imaging agent for NETs.

Other interesting tracers are [99m]Tc-demotate, with preliminary results in the preclinical and clinical setting,[30,31] and [111]In-DOTA-lanreotide ([111]In-DOTA-LAN, MAURITIUS [Multicenter Analysis of a Universal Receptor Imaging and Treatment Initiative: a European Study]), synthesized after the introduction of the macrocyclic chelator DOTA instead of DTPA.[32]

The radiopharmaceuticals are summarized in **Table 2**.[33,34]

## IMAGING TECHNIQUE

Guidelines for the scintigraphic imaging of NETs with [131/123]I-mIBG[35] and with [111]In-pentetreotide (SS receptor scintigraphy [SRS]) have been published in the United States[36] and Europe.[37]

Here, the essential steps to perform these examinations are outlined:

- Imaging request and justification of the examination: clinical indications
- Precaution before undertaking the examination/preparation of the patient and recommendations
- Radiopharmaceutical injection and recommendation after tracer administration

**Table 2**
**SS receptor radiopharmaceuticals**

| Full Name | Abbreviation |
|---|---|
| [123]I-Tyr3-octreotide | |
| [111]In-DTPA-D-Phe1-octreotide | [111]In-DTPA-OCT ([111]In-pentreotide) |
| [111]In-DOTA-D-Phe1-Tyr3-octreotide | [111]In-DOTA-TOC |
| [111]In-DOTA-Tyr3-octreotate | [111]In-DOTA-TATE |
| [111]In-DOTA-Nal3-octreotide | [111]In-DOTA-NOC |
| [111]In-DOTA-Nal3-Thr8-octrotide | [111]In-DOTANOC-ATE |
| [111]In-DOTA-Bz-Thi3-Thr8-octreotide | [111]In-DOTABOC-ATE |
| [99m]Tc-EDDA/HYNIC-Tyr3-octreotide | [99m]Tc-EDDA/HYNIC-TOC |
| [99m]Tc-EDDA/HYNIC-Tyr3-octreotate | [99m]Tc-EDDA/HYNIC-TATE |
| [123]I-Mtr-TOCA-octreotate | |
| [99m]Tc-demotate | |
| [111]In-DOTA-lanreotide | [111]In-DOTA-LAN (MAURITIUS) |
| [99m]Tc-depreotide | |
| [99m]Tc-vapreotide | |

- Imaging acquisition

## mIBG Scintigraphy

### Clinical indications

The request for mIBG scintigraphy usually arises for detection, staging, and restaging of primary NETs and their metastases, in case of pheochromocytomas, ganglioblastomas/neuroblastomas, paragangliomas, MEN2 syndrome, medullary thyroid carcinoma, and Merkel cell carcinoma.

This imaging technique is also used to select patients for therapy with $^{131}$I-mIBG and evaluate treatment response and follow-up. There are some nononcologic indications. such as the study of myocardial innervation and the functional evaluation of hyperplastic adrenals (**Box 1**).

### Precaution before examining/preparing the patient and recommendations

An absolute contraindication is pregnancy (confirmed or suspected).

Caution must be used in women who are breastfeeding: it should be interrupted for 48 hours after the examination when $^{123}$I is applied; it must be stopped if $^{131}$I is applied. Discontinuation of medications that could interfere with mIBG must be discussed with the referring physician (a detailed list of drugs interacting with mIBG is reported in the procedural guidelines issued by the European Association of Nuclear Medicine).

Preparation of the patient

- Thyroid blockade is essential to avoid thyroid irradiation from iodine. The administration of lugol solution or potassium iodide should start 1 day before the administration of radioiodinated mIBG and should continue after that for 1 to 4 days, depending on the use of $^{123}$I or $^{131}$I.
- Increase fluid intake to improve excretion of the radiopharmaceutical.
- Clear information about the examination and the use of radioactivity.

---

> **Box 1**
> **Clinical indications for $^{123/131}$I-mIBG scintigraphy in NETs**
>
> Detection of primary tumors and metastatic sites (staging and restaging)
>
> Detect relapse or progression of disease (follow-up in patients with known NET)
>
> Monitor the effects of treatment (surgery, chemotherapy, or radiotherapy)
>
> Select patients for radiometabolic treatment with $^{131}$I-mIBG

---

- Take detailed history about the tumor, information about recent laboratory or radiologic findings, previous treatments (radiometabolic therapy, chemotherapy, radiotherapy, or surgical).

Patients undergoing mIBG scintigraphy are often of pediatric age and therefore need particular attention and skilled staff.

### Radiopharmaceutical injection and recommendation after the tracer administration

Both $^{123}$I-mIBG and $^{131}$I-mIBG must be prepared according to the manufacturer's indications and, of course, quality control is needed before the intravenous injection. The administration is usually slow, over at least 5 minutes.

The suggested procedure for adults ranges between 40 and 80 MBq of $^{131}$I and is about 400 MBq for $^{123}$I. As in children, the procedure should be reduced according to the weight of the patient.

The radiation dosimetry varies depending on the isotope used. Patients are asked to void before images are acquired. After the examination, good hydration is recommended to improve the excretion of the tracer.

Radiation protection recommendations are given to the patient when discharged.

### Imaging acquisition

A single-head or multiple-head $\gamma$ camera is needed, and computed tomographic (CT) fusion, when available, should be implemented to improve the quality of the imaging.

Different collimators are necessary according to the isotope used. For $^{131}$I, a high-energy parallel hole is recommended, whereas for $^{123}$I, low-energy high resolution is recommended.

Planar and single-photon emission computed tomography (SPECT) images are acquired with different timing: at 24 hours for $^{123}$I, at 24 hours, 48 hours, and even later for $^{131}$I. Dedicated spot images may be useful to further investigate some areas of interest.

The imaging protocol can be summarized as follows:

- Preset energy settings for the heads of the camera according to the radioisotope in use
- Whole-body scan: for $^{131}$I-mIBG scanning speed of 4 cm/min; for $^{123}$I-mIBG, a scanning speed of 5 cm/min
- Planar spot as needed can be acquired with a 256 × 256 word matrix
- SPECT imaging of the appropriate regions, as indicated based on the clinical history; total number of projections, 120; 25 to 30 seconds per step; 128 × 128 word matrix

- Imaging processing and single-photon emission tomography (SPET) reconstruction

## SRS

### Clinical indications
The main clinical indications for scintigraphy in NETs, highlighted in **Box 2**, are staging, restaging, and follow-up of disease and selection of patients for peptide radioreceptor therapy (PRRT).[38]

Requests for imaging are mainly for NETs arising from the gastroenteropancreatic (GEP) tract, such as gastrinoma, insulinoma, and glucagonoma; from the lungs; from the skin as Merkel cell tumors; from the sympathoadrenal system, including pheochromocytoma, neuroblastoma, ganglioneuroma, and paraganglioma.

### Precaution before undertaking the examination/preparation of the patient and recommendations
An absolute contraindication is pregnancy (confirmed or suspected).

Relative contraindications are

- Breastfeeding
- Age younger than 18 years
- Clinically significant renal impairment (in consideration of the renal clearance of the tracer)
- Recent administration of cold SS analogue (this treatment should be stopped before imaging, but this issue is still a matter of debate)

Preparation of the patient

- Clear information about the examination and the use of radioactivity
- Take detailed history about the tumor, information about recent laboratory or radiologic findings, previous treatments (PRRT, chemotherapy, radiotherapy, or surgical)

---

**Box 2**
**Clinical indications for [111]In-pentetreotide scintigraphy in NETs**

Detection of primary tumors and of metastatic sites (staging and restaging)

Detect relapse or progression of disease (follow-up in patients with known NET)

Predict response to therapy (prognostic evaluation)

Monitor the effects of treatment (surgery, chemotherapy, or radiotherapy)

Select patients for PRRT

---

- Increase the fluid intake to improve renal excretion
- Some laxatives may be recommended in the days before imaging to reduce nonspecific tracer uptake in the bowel
- No need for fasting before injection

### Radiopharmaceutical injection and recommendation after tracer administration
[111]In-Pentetreotide is prepared according to the manufacturer's indications. After undergoing quality control, it is administered as an intravenous injection.

There is a range of the level of activity to be administered for imaging reported in the literature: from 120 to 220 MBq, and the recommended activity for good imaging quality is about 200 MBq.[37]

The radiation dosimetry is shown in **Table 3**.[36]

Patients are asked to void before images are acquired. After examination, good hydration is recommended to improve the excretion of the tracer. When returning home, patients should follow some radiation protection recommendations, including keeping distance from pregnant women and children.

### Imaging acquisition
A $\gamma$ camera equipped with a medium-energy parallel-hole collimator is needed. The correct setting requires [111]In photopeaks with a 20% window. Planar and SPECT images are acquired at 4 and 24 hours, sometimes up to 48 hours after injection (when the activity in the bowel is still significant at 24 hours).

The imaging protocol may be listed as follows:

- Preset energy settings for both heads of the camera: 172 and 254 keV with 20% window
- Whole-body scan: maximum scanning speed of 3 cm/min; a whole-body image may substitute for anterior and posterior spot images, with lower sensitivity to detect lesions
- Planar spot views of the head, chest, abdomen, pelvis, and, if needed, the extremities can be acquired for 10 to 15 min/image, using a 512 × 512 word matrix or 256 × 256 word matrix
- SPECT imaging of the appropriate regions, as indicated based on the clinical history; 360° of rotation; total number of projections, 120; 45 seconds per projection; 64 × 64 word matrix
- Imaging processing and SPET reconstruction

## IMAGING FINDINGS

Images obtained are analyzed and interpreted by a nuclear medicine physician.

**Table 3**
**Radiation dosimetry of $^{111}$In-pentetreotide administration in adults**

| Radiopharmaceutical | Administered Activity (MBq) | Organ Receiving the Largest Dose (mGy/MBq) | Effective Dose Equivalent (mSv/MBq) |
|---|---|---|---|
| $^{111}$In-Pentetreotide | 222 | Spleen 0.665 | 0.117 |

As discussed in the clinical indication section, mIBG scintigraphy is mainly requested to investigate pheochromocytomas, ganglioblastomas/neuroblastomas, paragangliomas, MEN2 syndrome, medullary thyroid carcinoma, and Merkel cell carcinoma, whereas SRS has a major role in the study of GEP NETs and lung carcinoids, with some applications also in pheochromocytomas, paragangliomas, medullary thyroid carcinoma, and Merkel cell carcinoma (**Table 4**).

Diagnostic criteria

- Knowledge of normal tissue uptake
- Clinical issue raised in the request for imaging
- History of the patient and clinical correlation with any other data from previous relevant examinations
- Intensity of the tracer uptake (a semiquantitative analysis of lesions may be useful in some cases)
- Knowledge of the cause of false-positive and false-negative images

In carcinoids, Modlin and colleagues[39] reported a 50% median detection rate and 76% sensitivity of mIBG scintigraphy; whereas a sensitivity of 84% has been shown for SRS.[40] However, mIBG can also show some uptake in nonoctreotide-avid lesions,[41] and it could play a complementary role in NET imaging, because its use in combination with SRS has been shown to increase sensitivity up to 95%.[42] Moreover, in 1 study, different metastases in the same patient were found with differential mIBG and SS analogue uptake.[43]

The overall results from the literature show that, despite the lower accuracy for other NETs, mIBG scintigraphy has been shown to have 90% sensitivity and high specificity for chromaffin tumors, including pheochromocytomas, neuroblastomas, and paragangliomas.[44]

The SRS sensitivity for the detection of pheochromocytoma was reported to be comparable with that of mIBG in some studies, but the number of patients evaluated was too low for a reliable conclusion.[20]

Generally, the heterogeneity of NETs influences the imaging results, and, therefore, they are discussed according to a clinical framework.

## GEP NETs

GEP tumors arise from the stomach, pancreas, and bowel, with a wide range of clinical features. The primary treatment in many cases is surgical, but any therapeutic decision cannot disregard the imaging work-up of these tumors, either in staging and restaging or during follow-up.

More experience with SRS has been reported for these tumors than with mIBG; however, both techniques have been applied in the past. It is only recently that the introduction of $^{68}$Ga-DOTA-peptide conjugate radiopharmaceuticals overcame SRS and mIBG.

There is a consolidated experience on the use of SRS in GEP, particularly its usefulness in detecting small lesions of the small bowel that are difficult to identify on conventional imaging with a sensitivity of 80% to 100% in localizing the primary tumor and disease burden,[45] which accounts for its success over the years (**Fig. 1**).

SPECT imaging can improve the detection of lesions, and these images might be requested for a more accurate evaluation.

In a large multicenter study including 253 patients affected by GEPs,[46] 82% diagnostic accuracy of SRS was obtained for abdominal sites of primary tumors. Other accuracy data were 94% for liver lesions, 91% for soft tissue lesions, and 98% for bone metastases.

**Table 4**
**Clinical applications of mIBG and SRS**

| | $^{131/123}$I-mIBG | SRS |
|---|---|---|
| GEP NETs | ± | + + |
| NETs of the lung | – – | + + |
| Pheochromocytoma paraganglioma | + + | ± |
| Neuroblastoma | + + | – – |
| Medullary thyroid carcinoma | + | + – |
| Merkel cell carcinoma | + | + – |
| Thymic carcinoids | + – | + – |
| Pituitary | – – | + – |

**A**                                    **B**

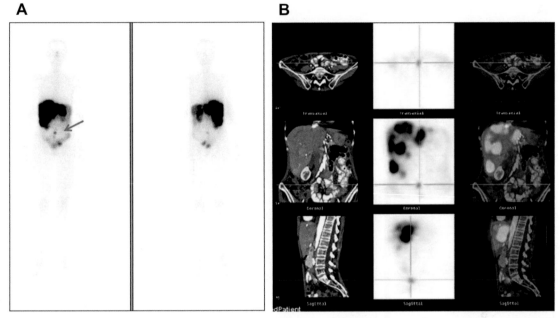

Fig. 1. SRS scan in a patient with liver metastases compatible with NET from an unknown primary. (*A*) Whole-body scan. (*B*) SPET/CT of the abdomen. Scintigraphic findings show the presence of a primary lesion in the small bowel (*red arrow*) and confirm multiple hepatic metastases.

Malignant islet cell tumors are named after their hormonal secretion: gastrinomas, vipomas, gluca-gonomas, and insulinomas, even although in 15% of cases, their presence is not related to a hypersecretive syndrome. The reported sensitivity of SRS is high, varying between 70% and 90%, although the sensitivity for insulinomas is generally lower, ranging between 20% and 60%.[47,48]

Another multicenter trial in Europe on histologically or biochemically proved neuroendocrine pancreatic tumors showed promising results, with a detection rate of 100% for glucagonomas, 88% for vipomas, 72% for gastrinomas, 82% for nonfunctioning islet cell tumors, and 87% for other carcinoids (**Fig. 2**).[49]

SRS has been widely adopted for diagnosis and also for clinical management in the restaging after surgery to assess the response to therapy and to plan further treatments.

Moreover, the detection of unknown and unexpected sites of diseases, not found at other imaging modalities, helps in modifying the therapeutic strategy in the management of the patient.[50]

A significant uptake is mandatory either for SS analogue therapy or for PRRT. The intense receptor expression seems to be associated with cellular differentiation and can be considered a prognostic factor, because poorly differentiated (and clinically more aggressive) neoplasias do not show significant radiolabeled SS analogue

uptake. In these cases, [$^{18}$F]fluorodeoxyglucose ($^{18}$F-FDG) uptake has been described as a measure of clinical aggressiveness.[51]

There is general agreement on the complementary role of $^{131}$I-mIBG /$^{123}$I-mIBG scintigraphy in GEPs, because some lesions that do not take up the radiolabeled SS analogue might be detected by mIBG.[41]

## NETs of the Lung

There is a spectrum of NETs of the lung ranging from well-differentiated bronchial NETs to highly malignant and poorly differentiated small-cell lung cancer (SCLC) and large-cell neuroendocrine carcinoma. The incidence is low, although it is reported to have increased over the past 30 years.[52]

SS receptors have been shown in most bronchial NETs, and several studies have assessed the diagnostic value of SRS. In a multicentric study by Reisinger and colleagues,[53] $^{111}$In-pentreotide scintigraphy yielded a sensitivity of 96% in diagnosing the primary tumor; sensitivity for detecting regional metastases was 60%, and 45% for distant metastases.

There is agreement about the high detection rate of lesions with SRS especially in SCLC, with a sensitivity up to 95% for the primary lesions[54] and an average reported sensitivity of 59% for metastases.

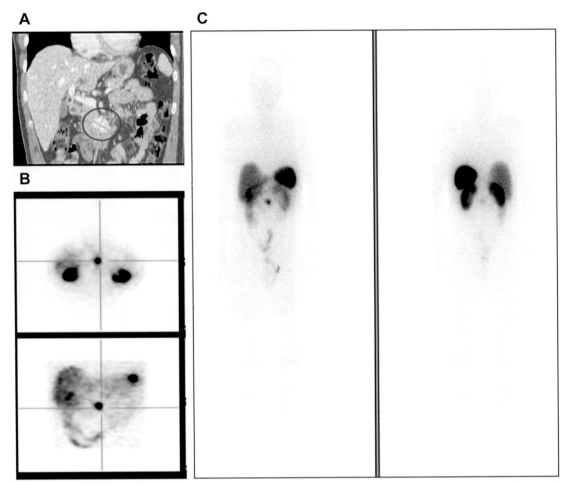

**Fig. 2.** Patient affected by a neuroendocrine tumor of the pancreas. (*A*) CT finding. The *red circle* indicates the primary pancreatic tumor. (*B*) Axial and coronal images of the scintigraphic uptake of the lesion. (*C*) Whole-body scan. [111]In-SRS evaluation confirmed pathologic uptake in the pancreatic region. No unexpected sites of diseases were shown.

Despite the limited sensitivity in the detection of distant metastases, SRS is useful in evaluating the extent of disease, because it is able to distinguish limited and extensive disease status, which is clinically relevant for treatment.

Among the tracers used for SS receptor imaging, [99m]Tc-depreotide is approved specifically for lung nodules and has been reported to have a sensitivity of 97% and a specificity of 73%.[55]

mIBG scintigraphy has no clinical role in the management of lung neuroendocrine cancer.

### Pheochromocytoma and Paraganglioma

Pheochromocytomas and paragangliomas share the sympathoadrenal lineage and are usually referred to as pheochromocytomas when arising from the adrenal glands and as paragangliomas when originating from aorticosympathetic paraganglia, including the organs of Zuckerkandl. Paragangliomas in the head and neck region are more often of parasympathetic origin and usually do not produce catecholamines.

Mostly sporadic, these tumors can be hereditary as well.

The malignancy of paragangliomas is not defined histologically but from the presence of metastases, and, therefore, proper imaging is mandatory to stage the disease correctly.

The major experience with both pheochromocytomas and paragangliomas is with mIBG scintigraphy, because mIBG is considered the prototypical tracer for studying these diseases (**Fig. 3**).

The overall sensitivity reported in the literature is 85% and the specificity is 89%,[56,57] and there are data on the superiority of [123]I-mIBG versus [131]I-mIBG.

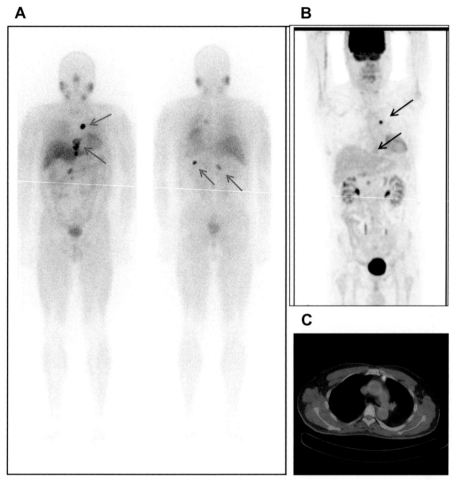

Fig. 3. Patient affected by pheochromocytoma. (*A*) Whole-body images (anterior and posterior view) with [123]ImIBG, showing multiple foci of pathologic uptake (*red arrows*); (*B, C*) [18]F-FDG-PET/CT (maximum intensity projection image, fused axial image) showing only the mediastinal lymphadenopathy (*black arrow*). Other lesions are not glucose avid, being well differentiated.

SRS sensitivity in these neoplasms has been reported as similar to that of mIBG scintigraphy, especially in the malignant forms, whereas the sensitivity reported for benign forms seems to be lower, ranging around 28.5% (**Fig. 4**).[57] However, the major drawback of receptor imaging is renal excretion, which makes the study of adrenal lesions more difficult.

In the evaluation of head and neck paragangliomas, SRS seems to have a greater role than mIBG, as reported by several studies.[58,59]

## Neuroblastoma

Neuroblastomas are highly malignant tumors of the neural crest, occurring in 97% of cases in children less than 10 years of age, representing the second most common solid malignancy in childhood.[60]

mIBG scintigraphy has been established in a large series of young patients, and is the most sensitive imaging technique, with a cumulative sensitivity of 92% and a specificity of nearly 100%.[61] Moreover, it is capable of identifying the presence of metastases, which is essential prognostic information (**Fig. 5**). Thus, mIBG scintigraphy is useful not only for primary diagnosis and staging but also to monitor treatment response and plan nuclear medicine therapy. The increased tumor/nontumor ratio of mIBG uptake, together with the long half-life of [131]I, is the basis for the therapeutic use of high activities of [131]I-mIBG.

SRS has not achieved a significant clinical role in the work-up of neuroblastoma, although a concordance of SRS and mIBG scintigraphy of about 85% has been reported, and there is some evidence that the presence of SS receptors in vitro in neuroblastoma correlates with a better prognosis and negativity to SS receptors could be related to a worse prognosis.[62]

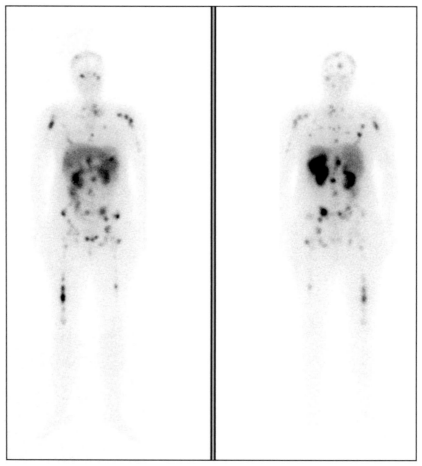

Fig. 4. Diffused skeletal involvement in a patient with metastatic pheochromocytoma, as shown by SRS whole-body images (anterior and posterior views).

## Medullary Thyroid Carcinoma

Medullary thyroid cancer arises from the parafollicular C cells and may be associated with MEN2A or MEN2B. The diagnostic role of mIBG scintigraphy has been evaluated in some studies, and the greatest sensitivity reported accounted for 41% with [123]I-mIBG in the detection of recurrent disease after surgery.[63] mIBG is applied only to identify patients who could benefit from [131]I-mIBG treatment. Similarly, SRS does not show high sensitivity, and both imaging techniques should not be relied on for either the initial diagnosis of medullary thyroid carcinoma or to exclude the disease (Fig. 6).

## Merkel Cell Carcinoma

Merkel cell carcinoma is a clinically aggressive, malignant neuroendocrine tumor of the skin, which has often already metastasized before the diagnosis. For this reason, FDG-PET/CT has been

evaluated as the imaging modality of choice for this kind of disease. However, there are few data on the possible role of mIBG and SRS. There are case reports about mIBG uptake in Merkel cell carcinoma.[64]

The experience with SRS is greater than with mIBG, but the results are limited.

Guitera-Rovel and colleagues[65] reported a sensitivity of 78% and a specificity of 96% with SRS in a series of 20 patients.

## Thymic Carcinoids

NETs of the thymus derive from Kulchitsky cells and are rare[66] and may be part of the clinical presentation in MEN1 syndrome.

There are few data regarding mIBG scintigraphy in this group of tumors[67] but the results are comparable with other carcinoids.

Gibril and colleagues[68] evaluated the role of SRS for NETs of the thymus compared with conventional

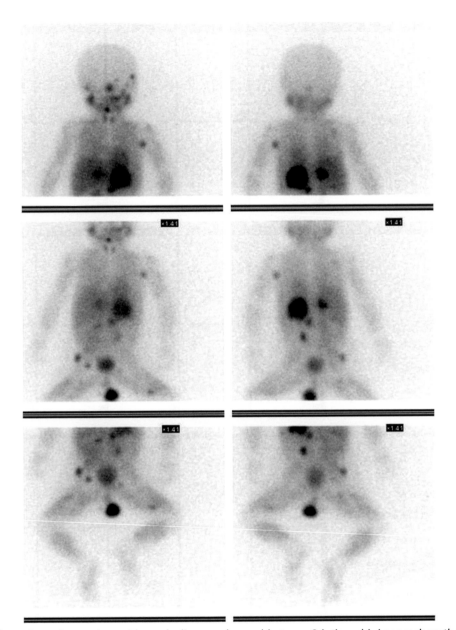

**Fig. 5.** $^{123}$I-mIBG scan in a patient with newly diagnosed neuroblastoma. Scintigraphic images show the presence of an abdominal mass, axillary lymphadenopathy, and diffused subcutaneous disease.

imaging and found that CT and magnetic resonance imaging were superior to SS receptor imaging.

### Pituitary

Pituitary adenomas, especially those producing growth hormone or thyroid-stimulating hormone, express SS receptors, showing some uptake in SRS, which is higher in functioning than in nonfunctioning lesions.[69,70]

However, physiologic uptake in the sellar region should be considered as a factor that decreases diagnostic accuracy.

### Differential Diagnosis, Pitfalls

Knowing the physiologic distribution of the tracer used for imaging is essential to detect areas of pathologic uptake. However, sources of error do exist.

In mIBG scintigraphy, for example, if the dimensions of the lesions are close or inferior to the spatial resolution of the γ camera, they might be missed, as well as those located next to areas of normal uptake.

Generally, errors in describing an mIBG scan may be related to

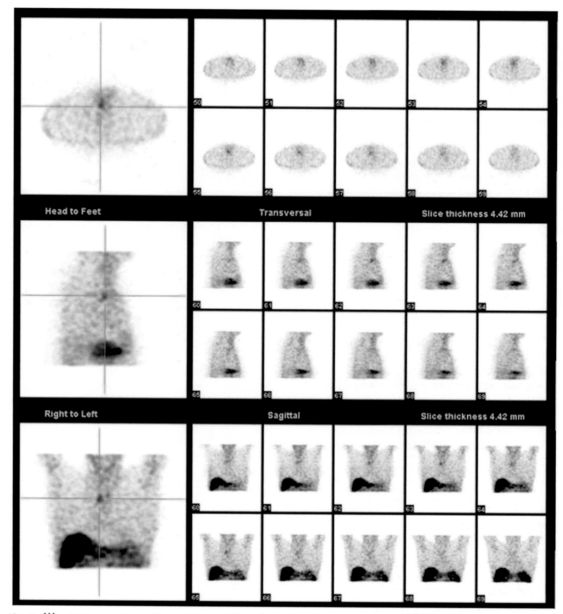

**Fig. 6.** [111]In-SRS in a patient affected by medullary thyroid carcinoma. Axial, sagittal, and coronal series showing pathologic uptake in the upper mediastinum compatible with nodal involvement.

- Specific features of the lesions (the dimension or the position close to foci of normal uptake, as discussed earlier, or a change in differentiation that prevents uptake of the tracer)
- Incorrect preparation for the examination (no thyroid blockade, not voiding before scanning, drug interference)
- Problems at the scanning procedure (movements of the patient, urine contamination)

- Normal variant, such as bilateral adrenal increased uptake, which can mask pathologic uptake

When reporting SRS, a differential diagnosis has to be considered for

- Nonneoplastic diseases and autoimmune disorders[71,72]
- Postradiation inflammatory disease
- Some bacterial infections

Imaging pitfalls are also possible. Common sources of misinterpretation are the presence of an accessory spleen, gallbladder uptake, urine contamination, pneumonitis, nasal uptake (paraphysiologic change during a cold), granulomatous disease.

Ongoing treatment with SS analogues (cold octreotide) may reduce uptake in the tumor site or reduce normal uptake in the liver and spleen.

The tumor itself could produce SS, which could compete with the tracer, resulting in a lower uptake in the lesions.

The presence of a different ssrt subtype with a lower affinity for the tracer (as in medullar thyroid cancer) may compromise the result of the SRS (Table 5).[73]

## APPENDIX

Other radiopharmaceuticals that are not commonly used for SPECT imaging of NETs include the following.

$^{99m}$Tc-(V)-Dimercaptosuccinic acid is a molecule that is actively taken up by the neoplastic cells because of their higher phosphate uptake. This radiopharmaceutical is used to study phosphate metabolism and has been applied mainly to medullary thyroid cancer, with moderate results and an average sensitivity of 51%.[74,75]

On the receptor imaging side, experimental tracers include receptor imaging developed for vasoactive intestinal peptide, bombesin, cholecystokinin, and glucagonlike peptide.

Another experimental tracer is the $^{123}$I-IMT (L-3-$^{123}$I-$\alpha$-methyl-thyrosine) a large synthetic amino acid developed to study the transport capability of tumor cells via the large amino acid transport (LAT) system. The possible applications of this radiopharmaceutical rely on LAT2 overexpression in NETs; however, it is not widely available.[76]

## SUMMARY

NETs constitute a multisided complex world that has always been challenging for physicians. Different imaging strategies have been developed targeting the peculiar features of this group of rare diseases. Efforts have been made to study metabolic characteristics and receptor expression on the tumor surface, amassing strong expertise and knowledge over the last 3 decades, which is still increasing as a result of the implementation of fusion imaging and the development of more detailed positron emission tomography tracers for NETs. However, in many countries, scintigraphic study of NETs is still the most widely available and convenient clinical technique for evaluating patients suspected to have these tumors.

## REFERENCES

1. Modlin IM, Oberg K, Chung DC, et al. Gastroenteropancreatic neuroendocrine tumours. Lancet Oncol 2008;9:61–72.
2. Modlin IM, Shapiro MD, Kidd M, et al. Siegfried Oberndorfer and the evolution of carcinoid disease. Arch Surg 2007;142:187–97.
3. Vinik AI, Woltering EA, Warner RR, et al. NANETS consensus guidelines for the diagnosis of neuroendocrine tumor. Pancreas 2010;39:713–34.
4. Taal BG, Visser O. Epidemiology of neuroendocrine tumours. Neuroendocrinology 2004; 80(Suppl 1):3–7.
5. Reubi JC. Neuropeptide receptors in health and disease: the molecular basis for in vivo imaging. J Nucl Med 1995;36:1825–35.
6. Short JH, Darby TD. Sympathetic nervous system blocking agents. III. Derivatives of benzylguanidine. J Med Chem 1967;10:833–40.
7. Wieland DM, Wu JL, Brown LE, et al. Radiolabeled adrenergic neuron blocking agents: adrenomedullary imaging with [131I]iodobenzylguanidine. J Nucl Med 1980;21:349–53.
8. Sisson JC, Frager MS, Valk TW, et al. Scintigraphic localization of phaeochromocytoma. N Engl J Med 1981;305:12–7.

| Table 5 Sources of misinterpretation of SRS: pitfalls and pearls | |
|---|---|
| Normal findings and variants | Accessory spleen Gallbladder uptake Urine contamination |
| Nonneoplastic diseases and autoimmune disorders | Nasal uptake (during cold) Pneumonitis and some bacterial infections Granulomatous disease Postradiation inflammatory disease |
| Pharmacologic/ chemical disturbances | Treatment with cold octreotide: reduction of uptake in the tumor site or a reduction of normal uptake in liver and spleen Lower uptake in the lesions with production of SS from the tumor itself |
| Variants | Presence of different ssrt subtype with a lower affinity for the tracer |

9. McEwan AJ, Shapiro B, Sisson JC, et al. Radioiodobenzylguanidine for the scintigraphic location and therapy of adrenergic tumors. Semin Nucl Med 1985;5:132–53.

10. Kolby L, Bernhardt P, Levin-Jakobsen AM, et al. Uptake of metaiodobenzylguanidine in neuroendocrine tumours is mediated by vesicular monoamine transporters. Br J Cancer 2003;89:1383–8.

11. Sisson JC, Wieland DM. Radiolabeled metaiodobenzylguanidine: pharmacology and clinical studies. Am J Physiol Imaging 1986;1:96–103.

12. Brazeau P, Vale W, Burgus R, et al. Hypothalamic polypeptide that inhibits the secretion of immunoreactive pituitary growth hormone. Science 1973; 179:77–9.

13. Arnold R, Simon B, Wied M. Treatment of neuroendocrine GEP tumours with somatostatin analogues: a review. Digestion 2000;62(Suppl 1):84–91.

14. Volante M, Bozzalla-Cassione F, Papotti M. Somatostatin receptors and their interest in diagnostic pathology. Endocr Pathol 2004;15(4):275–92.

15. Patel YC, Murthy KK, Escher EE, et al. Mechanism of action of somatostatin: an overview of receptor function and studies of the molecular characterization and purification of somatostatin receptor proteins. Metabolism 1990;39:63–9.

16. Reubi JC. Peptide receptors as molecular targets for cancer diagnosis and therapy. Endocr Rev 2003;24:389–427.

17. Pangerl T, Peck-Radosavljevic M, Kaserer K, et al. Somatostatin (SST) and VIP receptor subtype gene expression in human tumors. Eur J Nucl Med 1997; 24:995A.

18. Krenning EP, Bakker WH, Breeman WA, et al. Localisation of endocrine-related tumours with radioiodinated analogue of somatostatin. Lancet 1989; 1:242–4.

19. Lamberts SW, Bakker WH, Reubi JC, et al. Somatostatin receptor imaging in the localization of endocrine tumors. N Engl J Med 1990;323: 1246–9.

20. Krenning EP, Kwekkeboom DJ, Bakker WH, et al. Somatostatin receptor scintigraphy with 111In-DTPA-D-Phe1- and 123I-Tyr3-octreotide: the Rotterdam experience with more than 1000 patients. Eur J Nucl Med 1993;20:716–31.

21. Raynor K, Lucki I, Reisine T. Somatostatin receptors in the nucleus accumbens selectively mediate the stimulatory effect of somatostatin on locomotor activity in rats. J Pharmacol Exp Ther 1993;265: 67–73.

22. Hoyer D, Bell GI, Berelowitz M, et al. Classification and nomenclature of somatostatin receptors. Trends Pharmacol Sci 1995;16:86–8.

23. Anthony LB, Martin W, Delbeke D, et al. Somatostatin receptor imaging: predictive and prognostic considerations. Digestion 1996;57(Suppl 1):50–3.

24. Krenning EP, Bakker WH, Kooij PP, et al. Somatostatin receptor scintigraphy with [111In-DTPA-D-Phe1]-octreotide in man: metabolism, dosimetry and comparison with [123I-Tyr-3-]-octreotide. J Nucl Med 1992;33:652–8.

25. Maina T, Stolz B, Albert R, et al. Synthesis, radiochemistry and biological evaluation of a new somatostatin analogue (SDZ 219-387) labelled with technetium-99m. Eur J Nucl Med 1994;21:437–44.

26. Blum JE, Handmaker H, Rinne NA. The utility of a somatostatin-type receptor binding peptide radiopharmaceutical (P829) in the evaluation of solitary pulmonary nodules. Chest 1999;115:224–32.

27. Lebtahi R, Le Cloirec J, Houzard C, et al. Detection of neuroendocrine tumors: 99mTc-P829 scintigraphy compared with 111In-pentetreotide scintigraphy. J Nucl Med 2002;43:889–95.

28. Cwikla JB, Mikolajczak R, Pawlak D, et al. Initial direct comparison of 99mTc-TOC and 99mTc-TATE in identifying sites of disease in patients with proven GEP NETs. J Nucl Med 2008;49: 1060–5.

29. Hubalewska-Dydejczyk A, Fross-Baron K, Mikolajczak R, et al. 99mTc-EDDA/HYNIC-octreotate scintigraphy, an efficient method for the detection and staging of carcinoid tumours: results of 3 years' experience. Eur J Nucl Med Mol Imaging 2006;33:1123–33.

30. Maina T, Nock BA, Cordopatis P, et al. [(99m)Tc] Demotate 2 in the detection of sst(2)-positive tumours: a preclinical comparison with [(111)In] DOTA-tate. Eur J Nucl Med Mol Imaging 2006; 33(7):831–40.

31. Decristoforo C, Maina T, Nock B, et al. 99mTc-Demotate 1: first data in tumour patients–results of a pilot/phase I study. Eur J Nucl Med Mol Imaging 2003;30:1211–9.

32. Virgolini I, Britton K, Buscombe J, et al. 111In- and 90Y-DOTA-Lanreotide: results and implications of the MAURITIUS trial. Semin Nucl Med 2002;32: 148–55.

33. Pepe G, Moncayo R, Bombardieri E, et al. Somatostatin receptor SPECT–review article. Eur J Nucl Med Mol Imaging 2012;39(Suppl 1):S41–51.

34. Ambrosini V, Melopeni F, Fanti S, et al. Radiopeptide imaging in Europe. J Nucl Med 2011; 52(Suppl 12):42S–55S.

35. Bombardieri E, Giammarile F, Aktolun C, et al. 131I/ 123IMetaiodobenzylguanidine (mIBG) scintigraphy: procedure guidelines for tumour imaging. Eur J Nucl Med Mol Imaging 2010;37:2436–46.

36. Balon E, Goldsmith SJ, Siegel BA, et al. Procedure guideline for somatostatin receptor scintigraphy with 111In-Pentetreotide. J Nucl Med 2001;42: 1134–8.

37. Bombardieri E, Ambrosini V, Aktolun C, et al. 111In-pentetreotide scintigraphy: procedure guidelines

for tumour imaging. Eur J Nucl Med Mol Imaging 2010;37:1441–8.

38. Gnanasegaran G, Kapse N, Buscombe JR. Recent trends in radionuclide imaging and targeted radionuclide therapy of neuroendocrine tumours [Review article]. Indian J Nucl Med 2005;20(3):55–66.

39. Modlin IM, Latich I, Zikusoka M, et al. Gastrointestinal carcinoids: the evolution of diagnostic strategies. J Clin Gastroenterol 2006;40:572–82.

40. Modlin IM, Kidd M, Latich I, et al. Current status of gastrointestinal carcinoids. Gastroenterology 2005; 128:1717–51.

41. Kaltsas GA, Mukherjee JJ, Grossman AB. The value of radiolabelled MIBG and octreotide in the diagnosis and management of neuroendocrine tumours. Ann Oncol 2001;12(Suppl 2):S47–50.

42. Taal BG, Hoefnagel CA, Valdes Olmos RA, et al. Combined diagnostic imaging with 131I-MIBG and 111In-pentetreotide in carcinoid tumours. Eur J Cancer 1996;32:1924–32.

43. Quigley AM, Buscombe JR, Shah T, et al. Intertumoural variability in functional imaging within patients suffering from neuroendocrine tumours. An observational, crosssectional study. Neuroendocrinology 2005;82:215–20.

44. Hoefnagel CA, Voute PA, de Kraker J, et al. Radionuclide diagnosis and therapy of neural crest tumours using iodine-131 metaiodobenzylguanidine. J Nucl Med 1987;28:308–14.

45. Briganti V, Matteini M, Ferri P. Octreoscan SPET evaluation in the diagnosis of pancreas neuroendocrine tumors. Cancer Biother Radiopharm 2001;16: 515–24.

46. Chiti A, Briganti V, Fanti S. Results and potential in neuroendocrine gastro-entero-pancreatic tumors. Q J Nucl Med 2000;44:42–9.

47. Schillaci O, Massa R, Scopinaro F. 111In-pentetreotide scintigraphy in the detection of insulinomas: importance of SPECT imaging. J Nucl Med 2000;41:459–62.

48. Vezzosi D, Bennet A, Rochaix P, et al. Octreotide in insulinoma patients: efficacy on hypoglycemia, relationships with OctreoScan scintigraphy and immunostaining with anti-sst2A and anti-sst5 antibodies. Eur J Endocrinol 2005;152:757–67.

49. Krenning EP, Kwekkeboom DJ, Pauwels S, et al. Somatostatin receptor scintigraphy. In: Freeman LM, editor. Nuclear medicine annual. New York: Lippincott Williams & Wilkins; 1995. p. 1–50.

50. Westlin J, Janson ET, Arnberg H, et al. Somatostatin receptor scintigraphy of carcinoid tumours using the [111In-DTPA-D-Phe1]-octreotide. Acta Oncol 1993;32:783–6.

51. Garin E, Le Jeune F, Devillers A, et al. Predictive value of 18F-FDG PET and somatostatin receptor scintigraphy in patients with metastatic endocrine tumors. J Nucl Med 2009;50(6):858–64.

52. Yao JC, Hassan M, Phan A, et al. One hundred years after 'carcinoid': epidemiology of and prognostic factors for neuroendocrine tumors in 35,825 cases in the United States. J Clin Oncol 2008;26(18): 3063–72.

53. Reisinger I, Bohuslavitzki KH, Brenner W, et al. Somatostatin receptor scintigraphy in small-cell lung cancer: results of a multicenter study. J Nucl Med 1998;39:224–7.

54. Bombardieri E, Crippa F, Cataldo I, et al. Somatostatin receptor imaging of small cell lung cancer (SCLC) by means of 111In-DTPA octreotide scintigraphy. Eur J Cancer 1995;31A:184–8.

55. Blum J, Handmaker H, Lister-James J, et al. A multicenter trial with a somatostatin analog (99m)Tc depreotide in the evaluation of solitary pulmonary nodules. Chest 2000;117:1232–8.

56. Miskulin J, Shulkin BL, Doherty GM, et al. Is preoperative iodine 123 meta-iodobenzylguanidine scintigraphy routinely necessary before initial adrenalectomy for pheochromocytoma? Surgery 2003;134:918–22.

57. Ilias I, Chen CC, Carrasquillo JA, et al. Comparison of 6-(18) F-fluorodopamine PET with I-123-metaiodobenzylguanidine and In-111-pentetreotide scintigraphy in localization of nonmetastatic and metastatic pheochromocytoma. J Nucl Med 2008; 49:1613–9.

58. Koopmans KP, Jager PL, Kema IP, et al. In-111-octreotide is superior to I-123-metaiodobenzylguanidine for scintigraphic detection of head and neck paragangliomas. J Nucl Med 2008;49:1232–7.

59. Bustillo A, Telischi F, Weed D, et al. Octreotide scintigraphy in the head and neck. Laryngoscope 2004;114:434–40.

60. Olshan AF, Bunin GR. Epidemiology of neuroblastoma. In: Brodeur GM, Sawada T, Tsuchida Y, et al, editors. Neuroblastoma. Amsterdam (The Netherlands): Elsevier; 2000. p. 33–9.

61. Hoefnagel CA, de Kraker J. Childhood neoplasia. In: Murray IP, Ell PJ, editors. Nuclear medicine in clinical diagnosis and treatment. 2nd edition. London: Churchill Livingstone; 1998.

62. Kropp J, Hofmann M, Bihl H. Comparison of MIBG and pentetreotide scintigraphy in children with neuroblastoma. Is the expression of somatostatin receptors a prognostic factor? Anticancer Res 1997;17(3B):1583–8.

63. Faggiano A, Grimaldi F, Pezzullo L, et al. Secretive and proliferative tumor profile helps to select the best imaging technique to identify postoperative persistent or relapsing medullary thyroid cancer. Endocr Relat Cancer 2009;16:225–31.

64. Castagnoli A, Biti G, De Cristofaro MT, et al. Merkel cell carcinoma and iodine-131 metaiodobenzylguanidine scan. Eur J Nucl Med 1992;19(10): 913–6.

65. Guitera-Rovel P, Lumbroso J, Gautier-Gougis MS, et al. Indium-111 octreotide scintigraphy of Merkel cell carcinomas and their metastases. Ann Oncol 2001;12:807–11.

66. Tiffet O, Nicholson AG, Ladas G, et al. A clinicopathologic study of 12 neuroendocrine tumors arising in the thymus. Chest 2003;124(1): 141–6.

67. Hirano T, Otake H, Watanabe N, et al. Presurgical diagnosis of a primary carcinoid tumor of the thymus with MIBG. J Nucl Med 1995;36: 2243–5.

68. Gibril F, Chen YJ, Schrump DS, et al. Prospective study of thymic carcinoids in patients with multiple endocrine neoplasia type 1. J Clin Endocrinol Metab 2003;88:1066–81.

69. Kwekkeboom DJ, de Herder WW, Krenning EP. Receptor imaging in the diagnosis and treatment of pituitary tumors. J Endocrinol Invest 1999;22: 80–8.

70. Duet M, Mundler O, Azjenberg C. Somatostatin receptor imaging in non-functioning pituitary adenomas: value of an uptake index. Eur J Nucl Med 1994;21:647–50.

71. Kwekkeboom DJ, Krenning EP, Kho GS, et al. Somatostatin receptor imaging in patients with sarcoidosis. Eur J Nucl Med 1998;25(9):1284–92.

72. Kwekkeboom DJ, Krenning EP. Radiolabeled somatostatin analog scintigraphy in oncology and immune diseases: an overview. Eur Radiol 1997; 7(7):1103–9.

73. Kwekkeboom DJ, Kam BL, van Essen M, et al. Somatostatin receptor-based imaging and therapy of gastroenteropancreatic neuroendocrine tumours. Endocr Relat Cancer 2010;17:R53–73.

74. Denoyer D, Perek N, Le Jeune N, et al. Evidence that 99mTc-(V)-DMSA uptake is mediated by NaPi cotransporter type III in tumour cell lines. Eur J Nucl Med Mol Imaging 2004;31(1):77–84.

75. Koopmans KP, Neels ON, Kema IP, et al. Molecular imaging in neuroendocrine tumors: molecular uptake mechanisms and clinical results. Crit Rev Oncol Hematol 2009;71(3):199–213.

76. Jager PL, Meijer WG, Kema IP, et al. L-3-[123I]Iodo-alpha-methyltyrosine scintigraphy in carcinoid tumors: correlation with biochemical activity and comparison with [111In-DTPA-D-Phe1]-octreotide imaging. J Nucl Med 2000;41(11):1793–800.

# $^{18}$F-Fluorodihydroxyphenylalanine in the Diagnosis of Neuroendocrine Tumors

Heikki Minn, MD, PhD[a,b,]*, Jukka Kemppainen, MD[b,c],
Saila Kauhanen, MD[d], Sarita Forsback, PhD[b],
Marko Seppänen, MD[b,c]

## KEYWORDS

- $^{18}$F-Fluorodihydroxyphenylalanine • Neuroendocrine tumor • PET/computed tomography
- Pheochromocytoma • Medullary thyroid cancer

## KEY POINTS

- $^{18}$F-Fluorodihydroxyphenylalanine (FDOPA) shows high sensitivity in detecting catecholaminergic tumors such as pheochromocytomas and paragangliomas, and is the preferred tracer for nuclear medicine imaging of medullary thyroid cancer (MTC).
- The strengths of FDOPA include high tumor-to-background contrast, ability to identify lesions with low somatostatin receptor density, and convenience in assessing patients with MEN-2 syndrome who are at risk of having both MTC and pheochromocytoma owing to their genetic predisposition.
- The triad of FDOPA, $^{18}$F-fluorodeoxyglucose, and $^{68}$Ga-labeled 1,4,7,10-tetraazacyclododecane-1,4,7,10-tetraacetic acid (DOTA) peptides forms the backbone of all clinical imaging of neuroendocrine tumors in institutions with PET/computed tomography capability.

## INTRODUCTION

The current choice of radionuclide techniques for the imaging of neuroendocrine tumors (NETs) has expanded over the last 10 years and requires careful knowledge about the known or presumed characteristics of the disease entity, including genomic features. Tracer selection must take account of subsequent management, for example, whether surgery or another local form of therapy is considered or whether the patient should be a candidate for peptide-based radiotherapy (PBRT). While imaging of somatostatin receptors is preferred in most cases, the use of $^{18}$F-fluorodihydroxyphenylalanine (FDOPA) retains its value in 2 important tumor groups: catecholaminergic tumors derived from chromaffin cells of the neural crest (pheochromocytoma, paraganglioma) and medullary thyroid cancer (MTC). Furthermore, FDOPA can be distributed from the site of production to remote hospitals, and is a viable option for general imaging of NETs in institutions that do not have access to $^{68}$Ga chemistry.

For radiochemical synthesis of FDOPA, both electrophilic and nucleophilic fluorination methods are applicable. Electrophilic fluorodestannylation[1] is widely used, rapid, and easily automated, but suffers from poor yield and low specific radioactivity.

[a] Department of Oncology and Radiotherapy, Turku University Hospital, PO Box 52, Turku 20521, Finland; [b] Turku PET Centre, Turku University Hospital, PO Box 52, Turku 20521, Finland; [c] Department of Clinical Physiology and Nuclear Medicine, Turku University Hospital, PO Box 52, Turku 20521, Finland; [d] Division of Digestive Surgery and Urology, Turku University Hospital, PO Box 52, Turku 20521, Finland
* Corresponding author. Department of Oncology and Radiotherapy, Turku University Hospital, PO Box 52, Turku 20521, Finland.
E-mail address: heminn@utu.fi

PET Clin 9 (2014) 27–36
http://dx.doi.org/10.1016/j.cpet.2013.08.013
1556-8598/14/$ – see front matter © 2014 Elsevier Inc. All rights reserved.

Recently the more complicated but higher-yielding nucleophilic approach has been used in commercial synthesis devices[2] with improvement in the availability of FDOPA for human studies. FDOPA has been registered for human use in several European countries since 2006.[3] It may be purchased from the radiopharmaceutical industry, which renders FDOPA PET/computed tomography (CT) the preferred tracer in clinical nuclear medicine departments with limited or absent resources in radiochemistry.

The mechanism of tracer uptake has been established, and is related to capacity of NETs to store and secrete biogenic amines and hormones.[4] However, uptake may not be directly related to the magnitude or presence of hormonal activity, and active transport of neutral amino acids via the sodium-independent system L is an important mechanism of uptake[5] even in the presence of endocrine symptomatology. To enhance signal-to-noise ratio, carbidopa is commonly administered prior to imaging to block decarboxylase activity, which converts FDOPA to [18]F-fluorodopamine.[4,6] The experience in the diagnosis of a variety of NETs covers the last 15 years, and is thus longer and wider than that of any of the 1,4,7,10-tetraaza-cyclododecane-1,4,7,10-tetraacetic acid (DOTA) peptides or [11]C-labeled compounds.[3] **Box 1** highlights key information about the practical use of FDOPA among the increased diversity of tracers available for PET and single-photon emission CT.

This article presents the authors' experience of cases whereby FDOPA shows compelling evidence of added value in the management of NETs. Given the heterogeneity of NETs in expression of somatostatin receptors and the variable affinity of different DOTA peptides to 5 subclasses of receptors, it is obvious that patients with unexpected negative findings on peptide-based imaging may benefit from FDOPA, especially if no indication of poor differentiation, oncogenic activation, or other aggressive behavior exists. If the latter 3 features predominate, the authors suggest that [18]F-fluorodeoxyglucose (FDG) imaging should be considered. For a comprehensive review of FDOPA imaging in comparison with alternative tracers the reader is referred to the recent article by Balogova and colleagues,[3] which covers all important studies in various forms of NETs. This review also covers studies on those special forms of NETs for which FDOPA is not recommended as the first-line PET tracer, such as Merkel cell carcinoma, small cell lung cancer, and bronchial carcinoids. It must be emphasized, however, that even for these tumors, in sporadic cases FDOPA imaging can be useful as a complementary imaging modality.

---

**Box 1**
**Pearls, pitfalls, and practical points in the use of FDOPA for the diagnosis of NET**

*Interpretative Pearls*

Wide clinical experience covering 10 to 15 years and all different forms of NET

High specific uptake based on active transport and intracellular storage

Somatostatin receptor density is not directly related to uptake

Low uptake in inflammatory cells

Superior sensitivity compared with somatostatin receptor scintigraphy

Hormonal activity is not necessary for positive uptake, although metabolic and endocrine activity appear to have a relationship

"One-stop-shop" for evaluation of patients with MEN-2 syndrome

*Interpretative Pitfalls*

Shows fewer lesions than [68]Ga-labeled DOTA peptides in the majority of gastroenteropancreatic NETs

Not applicable if peptide-based radiotherapy is considered

Low uptake in paragangliomas of patients harboring mutated succinate dehydrogenase subunit B (SDHB)

Low uptake in medullary thyroid cancer (MTC) in patients having serum calcitonin doubling time less than 24 months

Low uptake in poorly differentiated NETs

*Practical Points*

Dynamic imaging may be useful in evaluation of pancreatic islet cell tumors and neck in patients with MTC

Preinjection oral carbidopa may mask uptake in islet-cell tumors

On-site radiopharmaceutical production is not mandatory; commercial vendors are available in Europe

---

## IMAGING TECHNIQUE AND ANALYSIS

The whole-body technique used at the authors' institution has been described previously.[7] In brief, the patients fast at least 6 hours before tracer injection, and 150 mg of carbidopa is administered orally 30 minutes before injection to curb amino acid decarboxylase activity peripherally. However, it is controversial as to whether patients with a suspicion of pancreatic islet-cell tumor should receive carbidopa, and experience and institutional guidelines do not support carbidopa use in this patient group.[6] It is not necessary to withhold octreotide, diazoxide, or cortisone before PET/CT imaging, because no interaction between metabolic activity and timing of endocrine treatment has been demonstrated for FDOPA.[8] In cases where abdominal findings are important, the patient is prehydrated by being asked to drink 1 to 1.5 L of water about 1 hour before starting the acquisition.

The dose of FDOPA is approximately 250 to 370 MBq in adults and 3.7 MBq/kg in children, and emission images are acquired in 3 dimensions in the caudad-cephalad direction starting from mid-thigh 60 minutes from intravenous injection. In patients with a suspicion of islet-cell tumors, dynamic imaging of the pancreas starts immediately after injection to help visualize early focal activity in the pancreatic head (**Fig. 1**). A lesion, particularly in the head of the pancreas, could be missed because of physiologic activity in the biliary system if only late images are obtained. Similarly, there is

some evidence of improved metastatic lymph node detection in the neck if dynamic imaging is applied in patients with MTC.[3] Emission imaging is combined with preinjection low-dose whole-body CT typically at 80 mAs and 120 kV if the procedure does not include diagnostic CT. In the latter case, standard contrast media and a higher radiation dose are used. In adults, organs with high physiologic activity apart from the pancreas include the basal ganglia, gallbladder, kidneys, and urinary bladder. Physiologic but usually only moderately increased uptake can also be seen in adrenal glands, degenerative bone lesions, and growth-plate fractures in young children. A typical FDOPA PET/CT with 250-MBq injected dose and low-dose CT covering 7 bed positions would result in an effective dose of 10.5 mSv in an adult patient with the urinary bladder wall as critical organ.

Image analysis is straightforward while all focal uptake not related to physiologic activity may represent NET or its metastases. However, uptake

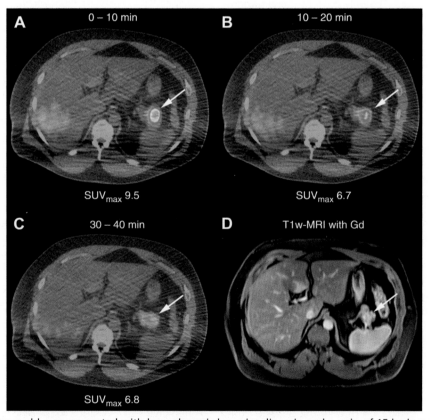

**Fig. 1.** A 48-year-old man presented with hypoglycemic hyperinsulinemia and a gain of 15 kg in weight during the last year. Dynamic FDOPA imaging of the pancreas over 60 minutes showed hypermetabolic focus in the caudal region (*arrow*), which was best visualized during the first 10 minutes (*A*), whereas later images between 10 and 20 minutes (*B*) and 30 and 40 minutes (*C*) show the lesion less conspicuously. Accordingly, the maximum standardized uptake value (SUV$_{max}$) is lower in the later phases of the acquisition. On gadolinium-enhanced T1-weighted magnetic resonance imaging (*D*), the lesion (*arrow*) measured 25 × 15 mm. The patient subsequently underwent resection of the pancreas, which confirmed the diagnosis.

without a clear anatomic counterpart, such as lymph node or bone or liver lesion, should be assessed with complementary techniques such as magnetic resonance (MR) imaging or bone scintigraphy in case of a potential therapeutic impact associated with the finding. In addition, it should be remembered that many FDOPA-positive skeletal metastases are not visualized on anatomic imaging, and histologic confirmation of all FDOPA-positive lesions is not feasible in most cases. Quantitative imaging using the maximum standardized uptake value ($SUV_{max}$) or its quotient may be helpful in monitoring treatment response or when total metabolic activity in all tumors is calculated.[9]

## GASTROENTEROPANCREATIC NEUROENDOCRINE TUMORS

Gastroenteropancreatic neuroendocrine tumors (GEP-NETs) are a mixed group of neoplasias sharing their origin in the neuroendocrine cells of the embryonic gut. Roughly 50% of these tumors arise from intestinal or gastric mucosa, and 30% originate in pancreatic endocrine cells.[10] While recognizing that [68]Ga-labeled octreotide analogues are preferred for evaluation of both hormonally active and silent GEP-NETs, especially when PBRT is considered, the authors emphasize that FDOPA is useful and a first option if [68]Ge/[68]Ga-generator and peptide-labeling synthesis devices are not available. Furthermore, in individual patients FDOPA has shown lesions that are negative on [68]Ga-octreotide, and further prospective comparative studies are warranted before the reciprocal superiority of these tracers can be determined in each clinical situation. For optimal surgery it might be necessary to perform both octreotide and FDOPA imaging if maximal cytoreduction with curative intent is the goal.

FDOPA is applicable for imaging of well or moderately differentiated GEP-NETs, especially if they originate from the midgut or pancreas. FDOPA is very useful in disclosing primary focus whenever a NET is suspected based on abnormal hormonal activity (**Fig. 2**). In the case of bronchial or hindgut NETs, the results are less satisfactory, and the authors recommend [68]Ga PET/CT with DOTA peptides or FDG PET/CT depending on the presumed malignancy grade of the tumor. In the compiled evaluation of different studies consisting of 76 patients having digestive carcinoid GEP-NETs, Balogova and colleagues[3] reported sensitivity of FDOPA imaging based on patient, site, and lesion to be 89%, 76%, and 97%, respectively. This result compares very favorably with that of somatostatin receptor scintigraphy,

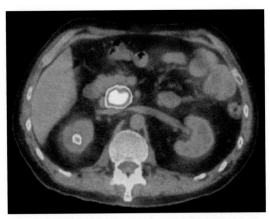

Fig. 2. A previously healthy 51-year-old man presented with ectopic secretion of corticotropin without clear confirmation of the site of hormonally active focus on anatomic imaging. FDOPA PET/CT showed a metabolically active tumor in contact with the pancreatic head and duodenum, and no distant metastatic lesions. At operation the tumor measured 4 cm, and showed typical neuroendocrine features and low proliferative activity. The patient remains free of disease 3.5 years after surgery, and follow-up FDOPA imaging is negative.

and is not decisively inferior to [68]Ga PET/CT with DOTA peptides. A patient with negative FDG and positive FDOPA PET/CT findings prior to radical surgery is presented in **Fig. 3**.

FDOPA uptake on PET was found to reflect metabolic endocrine activity and urinary 5-hydroxyindoleacetic acid, the main metabolite of serotonin, in 77 patients with mostly midgut GEP-NETs.[9] However, no association between FDOPA metabolic activity and the most important serum biomarker, chromogranin A, could be demonstrated. These investigators detected 979 FDOPA-positive lesions (median of 12 per patient) demonstrating the value of FDOPA for general assessment of metabolic tumor burden in widely disseminated GEP-NETs. Because [68]Ga PET/CT with DOTA peptides shows typically more lesions in GEP-NETs than does FDOPA, the authors hypothesize that the former tracer is better suited to assessment of total tumor burden.[11] Despite this, the authors have found FDOPA PET/CT to be useful for potentially operable patients with GEP-NETs of carcinoid type to assist in primary tumor localization and evaluation of small-volume metastatic disease (see **Fig. 3**).[12] A negative FDOPA study in these patients having anatomically defined tumors suggests that malignant differentiation and tumor load should then be evaluated with standard FDG PET/CT. Furthermore, patients with FDOPA-negative and FDG-positive metastases are less likely to benefit from debulking surgery and should be considered for

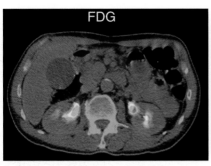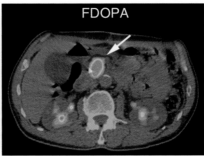

Fig. 3. Preoperative FDG and FDOPA axial PET/CT images of a 59-year-old man who received pancreaticoduode-nectomy because of a low-grade pancreatic GEP-NET metastasizing in multiple local lymph nodes. Note that FDG imaging was totally negative, whereas FDOPA imaging clearly showed tumor in the pancreatic head (*arrow*) and a nodal metastasis (not depicted here but seen in **Fig. 4A**).

adjunctive systemic treatment. Patients with negative FDG and positive FDOPA, in turn, typically enjoy a good prognosis despite the appearance of metastatic lesions, and may show durable response to endocrine therapy (**Fig. 4**).

Insulinomas and lesions with β-cell hyperplasia in the pancreas deserve special attention. If benign, these tumors can be cured by adequate surgery, and localization of hormonally active foci is of utmost importance. Preoperative FDOPA imaging of the focal form of neonatal hyperinsulinism allows noninvasive characterization of the lesion, which enables limited surgery and retention of the healthy parts of pancreas.[3,4,8] The authors' experience in FDOPA imaging of adult patients is more favorable than that of some other institutions (see **Fig. 1**), which may in part be explained by a preference not to give oral carbidopa before dynamic imaging of the pancreas.[6] This preference arises from the general observation of decreased uptake in pancreas after carbidopa premedication, which seems to affect the target cells even more and results in reduced signal-to-noise ratio.

## PHEOCHROMOCYTOMA AND PARAGANGLIOMA

Pheochromocytoma and paraganglioma represent uncommon tumors with variable, though usually low, malignant potential, but distinct endocrine activity and hereditary background in up to 30% of cases.[13] Their origin in chromaffin cells makes them susceptible to radioiodinated meta-iodobenzylguanidine (MIBG) treatment, and patients who are candidates for high doses of MIBG should first be evaluated with $^{123}$I-MIBG scintigraphy, which has sensitivity of more than 90% in detecting pheochromocytoma in meta-analytical evaluation under optimal circumstances.[14] Despite this high performance, all parallel comparisons between $^{123}$I-MIBG scintigraphy and FDOPA imaging

have indicated the latter to be more sensitive in detecting primary pheochromocytoma, and the authors' experience in staging and restaging yielded 100% sensitivity in 25 patients.[12] The authors consider FDOPA PET/CT to be useful for evaluating patients with a suspicion of pheochromocytoma based on serum or urinary catecholamine measurement and a known genetic syndrome such as multiple endocrine neoplasia type 2 (MEN-2). These patients are at risk for bilateral tumors, and sensitivity of standard CT or MR imaging is lower in comparison with sporadic cases that usually present unilaterally in adrenal medulla. In addition, FDOPA imaging is commonly recommended when there is suspicion of recurrent or metastatic pheochromocytoma (**Fig. 5**).

FDOPA PET/CT is useful if local therapy such as neck dissection or stereotactic irradiation is considered for treatment of paragangliomas in the head and neck area (**Fig. 6**). Indeed, a recent meta-analysis of 11 studies and 275 patients indicated pooled sensitivity of FDOPA PET and PET/CT in the diagnosis of head and neck paragangliomas to be 91% on a patient basis and 79% on a lesion basis, while specificity was 95% for both types of analyses.[15] FDOPA is suitable for imaging of adrenal, extra-adrenal, sympathetic, parasympathetic, functioning, nonfunctioning, metastatic, and non-metastatic paraganglioma.[3] These all-round features with relative insensitivity to individual tumor characteristics render FDOPA the tracer of choice for PET imaging of paragangliomas and pheochromocytomas, with the following important exception. Patients with a rare mutation in succinate dehydrogenase subunit B (SDHB) have typically FDOPA-negative tumors and should be imaged with FDG, which shows a satisfactory overall lesion-based sensitivity of 83% in detecting tumors harboring mutated SDHB (reviewed in Ref.[16]). Preference to glycolysis is a well-established hallmark of cancer; whenever aggressive growth dominates

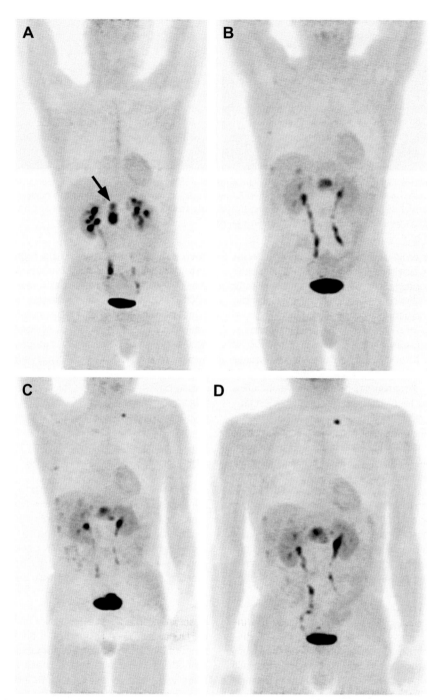

**Fig. 4.** Serial FDOPA PET/CT scans of the same patient illustrated in **Fig. 3**. The preoperative scan (*A*) shows only the primary lesion and nodal metastasis cranial from the primary (*arrow*), whereas the repeat scan 2 years after the operation (*B*) indicates dissemination of disease in liver and skeleton in an asymptomatic phase when serum chromogranin A started to increase. Note that the pancreatic bed at the level of right kidney pelvis is free of tumor in *B*. Subsequent FDOPA imaging (*C, D*) has demonstrated nodal metastasis in the left supraclavicular fossa, but the patient remains stable and in good health on octreotide treatment 6 years after the operation.

clinical presentation, FDG, rather than FDOPA to demonstrate a so-called flip-flop phenomenon,[16] should be considered for evaluation of paraganglio-mas even if SDHB status is unknown (see **Box 1**).

## MEDULLARY THYROID CANCER

MTC, which derives from the parafollicular C cells, is the least common of differentiated thyroid

**A**  PET/CT

**B**  PET

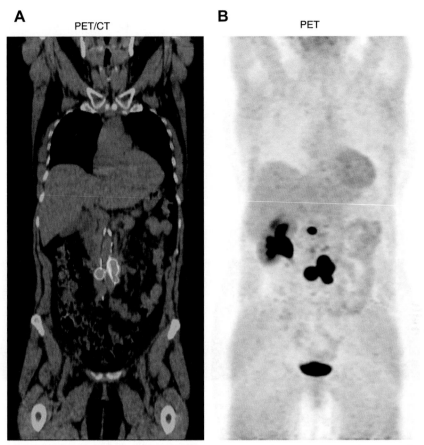

Fig. 5. FDOPA imaging in a 59-year-old woman who underwent left adrenalectomy because of a pheochromocytoma with uncertain malignant potential. Postoperatively urinary normetanephrines remained abnormal, and asymptomatic para-aortic lymph node metastases were found 8 months later on FDOPA PET/CT (*A*) and PET (*B*), indicating that the pheochromocytoma was malignant. Subsequently the patient received several courses of meta-iodobenzylguanidine (MIBG) and cytostatic therapy with modest response. The patient died 7.5 years after the primary operation.

cancers and comprises 3% to 5% of all thyroid malignancies. About 75% of cases are sporadic, and almost all of the remaining patients present with MEN-2 syndrome in which MTC is the most important neoplastic manifestation. All of the inherited cases and approximately 45% of the sporadic cases harbor an activation mutation in the RET proto-oncogene, which is caused by a germline change in MEN-2 and somatic change in sporadic MTC, respectively, on chromosome 10 (reviewed in Ref.[13]). Of interest is the recent advancement in treatment of locally advanced or metastatic MTC using targeted drugs that inhibit RET, such as vandetanib and cabozantinib.[17] The natural progression of MTC is usually slow, and patients may benefit from re-resection, external-beam radiotherapy, or tyrosine kinase inhibitors targeting RET in cases of suspicion or confirmation of recurrence or progression of disease. Both serum calcitonin and carcinoembryonic antigen

(CEA) are routine biomarkers during follow-up of patients with MTC, and metabolic imaging is used after thyroidectomy to assess resectability of metastases and general tumor load, and as an adjunct to serum biomarkers in response monitoring.

FDG and FDOPA PET/CT complement morphologic imaging by conferring prognostic information and by increasing sensitivity to detect unsuspected metastatic disease, especially in the neck. The pooled sensitivity, on both patient and lesion basis, of detecting MTC was 95% for FDOPA, whereas those for FDG were 44% and 42%, respectively.[3] Of all available PET tracers, including $^{68}$Ga-labeled DOTA peptides, FDOPA seems to be the tracer of choice when calcitonin and CEA doubling times are longer than 24 months, whereas patients with short calcitonin and CEA doubling times or initially high biomarker concentrations are likely to have a more aggressive disease and should be imaged with FDG or both tracers.[7,18]

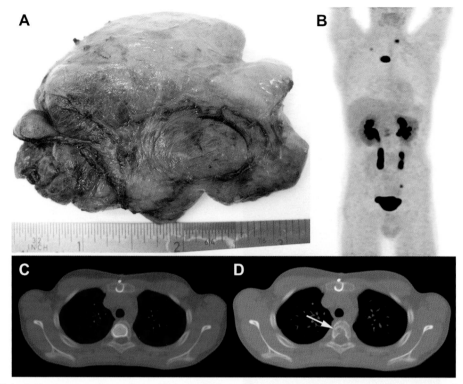

**Fig. 6.** Metastatic paraganglioma in a 15-year-old boy who presented with protracted growth, hypertonia, increased urinary catecholamine secretion, and left cervical adenopathy. The neck node, which measured 8 cm, was hyperemic, and first embolized and then operated on (*A*), which confirmed the diagnosis and showed on histopathologic examination low proliferative activity (Ki-67 2%) in neuroendocrine cells. Postoperative FDOPA PET/CT (*B–D*) revealed residual left neck node (*B*), right apical lung metastasis (*B*), and bone metastasis in fourth thoracic vertebra (*B, C*), which showed a small lytic component on anatomic CT (*D, arrow*). Both MIBG and somatostatin receptor scintigraphy were negative for lung and bone lesions, demonstrating the superior sensitivity of FDOPA in detecting metastatic paraganglioma. Postoperatively, endocrine activity has normalized, and follow-up FDOPA imaging has not shown progression of disease 1 year after surgery without any systemic treatment.

Because only one prospective trial comparing FDOPA and FDG in MTC appears to have been published,[7] it is difficult to state exact thresholds of serum tumor marker levels or doubling times for selection of the best tracer. Furthermore, in patients with long serum marker doubling times, negative findings on both FDOPA and FDG imaging are common, and these patients may be candidates for follow-up rather than for medical interventions. Because FDG and FDOPA may detect different lesions, their complementary role in difficult clinical situations (eg, in determination of the extent of neck dissection) should be considered. Balogova and colleagues[3] recommend FDOPA as the best tracer in cases with elevated tumor markers after thyroidectomy if the calcitonin level is higher than 150 ng/mL, and in their experience early image acquisition during the first 15 minutes is advised to help visualization of neck nodes. The authors also advocate FDOPA as the first-line PET study in MTC (**Fig. 7**), with the exception of patients showing symptoms or signs of rapidly

progressing disease including short calcitonin and CEA doubling times.[4,7] Both FDOPA and FDG positivity carry an inferior prognosis in comparison with PET-negative cases, with FDG showing stronger prognostic information.[18]

## SUMMARY

Despite the emerging role of [68]Ga-labeled DOTA peptides in the evaluation of different types of NETs, FDOPA seems to retain its value in certain patients for whom PET imaging is necessary. The cases favoring FDOPA include patients who have or are suspected of having a pheochromocytoma, paraganglioma, islet-cell tumor, and—as complement to [68]Ga-DOTA peptide imaging—carcinoid type of GEP-NET whereby the location of primary tumor is unknown. Patients with resected MTC showing elevated serum tumor markers are also strong candidates for FDOPA imaging.[7] The strengths of FDOPA include high tumor-to-background contrast, ability to identify lesions

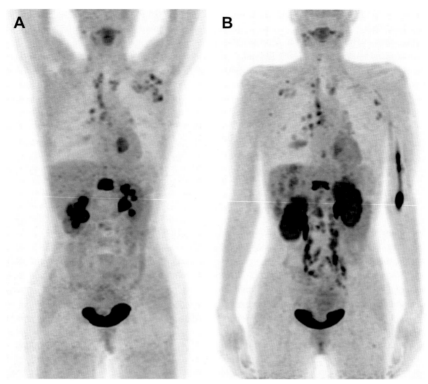

**Fig. 7.** This woman underwent thyroidectomy at 34 years of age because of a metastatic medullary thyroid cancer (MTC). No mutations in RET proto-oncogene suggestive of MEN-2A syndrome were detected, and the patient underwent multiple FDOPA PET/CT scans during follow-up and treatment of her metastatic MTC over 8 years. Comparison between scans *A* (October 2008) and *B* (January 2011) demonstrates progression of disease, notably in the liver, lungs, and lymph nodes, after sorafenib treatment lasting more than 2.5 years. The uptake in the left arm in *B* is due to partial extravasation of tracer.

with low somatostatin receptor density, and convenience in assessing patients with MEN-2 syndrome who are at risk of having both MTC and pheochromocytoma owing to their genetic predisposition. Furthermore, FDOPA is very rarely positive in inflammatory lesions,[3] and may be shipped to PET imaging facilities without cyclotrons. A related compound, [18]F-labeled dopamine, is available in a few dedicated centers, but is not easily produced or delivered to busy nuclear medicine units outside academic hospitals.[16] The triad of FDOPA, FDG, and [68]Ga-labeled DOTA peptides forms the backbone of all clinical NET imaging in institutions with PET/CT capability. The individual roles of the 3 tracers need to be seen as complementary, with information on patient and tumor characteristics, including association with genetic syndromes and specific mutations, determining the final choice.

## REFERENCES

1. Namavari M, Bishop A, Satymurthy N, et al. Regioselective radiofluorodestannylation with [[18]F]F2 and [[18]F]CH₃COOF: a high yield synthesis of 6-[[18]F]fluoro-L-dopa. Int J Rad Appl Instrum A 1992;43:989–96.

2. Libert LC, Frabci X, Plenevaux AR, et al. Production at the Curie level of no-carrier-added 6-[18]F-fluoro-L-dopa. J Nucl Med 2013;54(7):1154–61. http://dx.doi.org/10.2967/jnumed.112.112284.

3. Balogova S, Talbot JN, Nataf V, et al. [18]F-Fluorodihydroxyphenylalanine vs other radiophramaceuticals for imaging neuroendocrine tumours according to their type. Eur J Nucl Med Mol Imaging 2013;40:943–66.

4. Minn H, Kauhanen S, Seppänen M, et al. Focus on molecular imaging: [18]F-FDOPA—a multiple target molecule. J Nucl Med 2009;50:1915–8.

5. Crippa F, Alessi A, Serafini GL. PET with radiolabeled amino acids. Q J Nucl Med Mol Imaging 2012;56:151–62.

6. Kauhanen S, Seppänen M, Nuutila P. Premedication with carbidopa masks positive finding of insulinoma and β-cell hyperplasia in [18]F-dihydroxy-phenylalanine positron emission tomography. J Clin Oncol 2008;26:5307–8.

7. Kauhanen S, Schalin-Jäntti C, Seppänen M, et al. Complementary roles of [18]F-DOPA PET/CT and

$^{18}$F-FDG PET/CT in medullary thyroid cancer. J Nucl Med 2011;52:1855–63.

8. Arnoux JB, de Lonlay P, Ribeiro MJ, et al. Congenital hyperinsulinism. Early Hum Dev 2010;86:287–94.

9. Fiebrich HB, de Jong JR, Kema IP, et al. Total $^{18}$F-DOPA PET tumour uptake reflects metabolic endocrine tumour activity in patients with a carcinoid tumour. Eur J Nucl Med Mol Imaging 2012;38:1854–61.

10. Öberg K, Knigge U, Kwekkeboom D, et al. Neuroendocrine gastro-entero-pancreatic tumors: ESMO clinical practice guidelines for diagnosis, treatment and follow-up. Ann Oncol 2012;23(Suppl 7):vii124–30.

11. Ambrosini V, Tomasetti P, Castellucci P, et al. Comparison between $^{68}$Ga DOTA-NOC and $^{18}$F-DOPA PET for the detection of gastro-entero-pancreatic and lung neuro-endocrine tumors. Eur J Nucl Med Mol Imaging 2008;35:1431–8.

12. Kauhanen S, Seppänen M, Ovaska J, et al. The clinical value of [$^{18}$F]Fluorodihydroxyphenylalanine positron emission tomography in primary diagnosis, staging and restaging of neuroendocrine tumors. Endocr Relat Cancer 2009;16:255–65.

13. Strosberg JR. Update on the management of unusual neuroendocrine tumors: pheochromocytoma and paraganglioma, medullary thyroid cancer and adrenocortical carcinoma. Semin Oncol 2013;40:120–33.

14. Jacobson AF, Deng H, Lombard J, et al. $^{123}$I-meta-iodobenzylguanidine scintigraphy for the detection of neuroblastoma and pheochromocytoma: results of a meta-analysis. J Clin Endocrinol Metab 2010;95:2596–606.

15. Treglia G, Cocciolillo F, de Waure C, et al. Diagnostic performance of $^{18}$F-dihydroxyphenylalanine positron emission tomography in patients with paraganglioma: a meta-analysis. Eur J Nucl Med Mol Imaging 2012;39:1144–53.

16. Havekes B, King K, Lai EW, et al. New imaging approaches to pheochromocytomas and paragangliomas. Clin Endocrinol (Oxf) 2010;72:137–45.

17. Giunti S, Antonelli A, Amorosi A, et al. Cellular signalling pathway alterations and potential targeted therapies for medullary thyroid carcinoma. Int J Endocrinol 2013;2013:803171. http://dx.doi.org/10.1155/2013/803171.

18. Verbeek HH, Plukker JT, Koopmans KP, et al. Clinical relevance of $^{18}$F-FDG and $^{18}$F-DOPA PET in recurrent medullary thyroid carcinoma. J Nucl Med 2012;53:1863–71.

# $^{68}$Ga-DOTA-peptides in the Diagnosis of NET

Valentina Ambrosini, MD, PhD*, Stefano Fanti, MD

## KEYWORDS

- $^{68}$Ga-DOTA-peptides • PET/CT • Neuroendocrine tumors • Somatostatin receptors

## KEY POINTS

- $^{68}$Ga-DOTA-peptides are a group of radiopharmaceuticals that specifically bind to somatostatin receptors overexpressed on NET cells (with variable affinity).
- Currently there are no reports supporting the preferential use of one analogue (DOTA-TOC, DOTA-NOC, DOTA-TATE) over the other.
- $^{68}$Ga-DOTA-peptides are accurate for the detection of well-differentiated NET lesions at the primary and metastatic sites.
- PET/CT with $^{68}$Ga-DOTA-peptides has a relevant impact on patients' clinical management (in particular, regarding whether to initiate therapy with hot or cold somatostatin analogues and to guide the course of treatment) and provides prognostic information.
- Indications to study NET include staging and restaging, detection of the unknown primary tumor or of disease relapse, and follow-up.

The introduction in the clinic of somatostatin receptor scintigraphy (SRS) has represented a milestone in neuroendocrine tumor (NET) diagnostic imaging, with an overall detection rate of somatostatin receptor (SSR)–positive tumors[1] ranging between 80% and 100%. However, SRS presents some limitations including imaging organs with higher physiologic uptake (eg, liver); the detection of small lesions (because of suboptimal spatial resolution of the isotopes used for SPECT imaging)[2,3]; the relatively higher costs (compared with PET imaging); and the longer image acquisition protocol.

To overcome such limitations, new beta-emitting radiopharmaceuticals that specifically bind to SSR ($^{68}$Ga-DOTA-peptides) have been recently used as part of clinical trials in specialized centers in Europe. $^{68}$Ga-DOTA-peptides are a group of radiopharmaceuticals presenting a common structure:

a beta-emitting isotope ($^{68}$Ga); a chelant (DOTA); and the ligand of SSR (NOC, TOC, TATE). $^{68}$Ga-DOTA-peptides (DOTA-TOC, DOTA-NOC, DOTA-TATE) specifically bind to SSR-subtypes overexpressed on NET cells with variable affinity: all radiotracers can bind to SSR2 and to SSR5, whereas only $^{68}$Ga-DOTA-NOC also presents a good affinity for SSR3.[4–6]

The number of papers describing the results obtained with $^{68}$Ga-DOTA-peptides PET/CT in patients with NET has exponentially increased in the past few years. Although the first compound to be clinically used was DOTA-TOC, the use of DOTA-NOC and DOTA-TATE has significantly increased recently. The overall sensitivity and specificity for the detection of NET ranges between 90% and 98% and 92% and 98%, respectively.[7,8]

Current guidelines state that there is no evidence supporting the preferential use of one analogue

Conflict of Interest: The authors have nothing to disclose.
Nuclear Medicine, S.Orsola-Malpighi University Hospital, University of Bologna, Via Massarenti 9, Bologna 40138, Italy
* Corresponding author. Nuclear Medicine, Pad 30, S.Orsola-Malpighi University Hospital, Via Massarenti 9, Bologna 40138, Italy.
E-mail address: valentina.ambrosini@aosp.bo.it
PET Clin 9 (2014) 37–42
http://dx.doi.org/10.1016/j.cpet.2013.08.007

over the other,[9] and recent papers of comparison reported comparable diagnostic accuracy.[10,11] Factors in favor of the use of DOTA-NOC include the wider spectrum of SSR affinity and lower dosimetry, whereas DOTA-TOC and DOTA-TATE have the advantage that they can be used for diagnosis (if labeled with [68]Ga) and subsequent treatment (when labeled with [177]Lutetium or [90]Yttrium).

In all cases the synthesis and labeling process is easy and economic: gallium can be easily eluted from a commercially available Ge-68/Ga-68 generator and therefore there is no need of an on-site cyclotron. [68]Ga (t1/2 = 68 minutes) presents an 89% positron emission and negligible gamma emission (1077 keV) of 3.2%. The long half-life of the mother radionuclide [68]Ge (270.8 days) makes it possible to use the generator for approximately 9 to 12 months depending on the requirement, rendering the whole procedure relatively economic.[11] Another advantage of [68]Ga-peptides compared with metabolic tracers (eg,

[18]F-DOPA, [18]F-FDG) is that they provide data on receptors expression, particularly relevant before starting targeted nuclide therapy. Finally, compared with SRS, PET/CT is a single-day examination.

From a clinical point of view, [68]Ga-DOTA-peptides PET/CT is performed to image patients with NET for disease staging and restaging, follow-up, detection of unknown primary tumor sites, and selection of patients before starting therapy with either hot or cold somatostatin analogues.

[68]Ga-DOTA-peptides PET/CT has been proved an accurate procedure for the detection of primary and secondary NET lesions, with superior results to CT and SRS (**Fig. 1**). One of the studies with the largest populations (84 patients)[7] demonstrated that [68]Ga-DOTA-TOC PET/CT accuracy (96%) was significantly higher than that of CT (75%) and In-111 SRS-SPECT (58%). PET/CT was particularly accurate for the detection of lesions at node, bone, and liver level. Overall, PET/CT-derived data were relevant to change the patient's clinical management in 14% of the

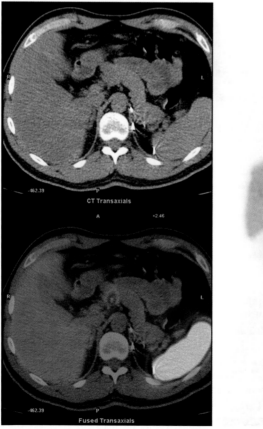
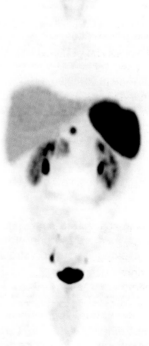

**Fig. 1.** [68]Ga-DOTA-NOC PET/CT transaxial and MIP images of a 38-year-old male patient with multiple endocrine neoplasia syndrome, previously operated for pheocromocytoma. PET/CT with [68]Ga-DOTA-NOC showed a focal and pathologic area of tracer uptake in the pancreatic body (SUVmax 23) undetected by other imaging procedures ([18]F-DOPA and morphologic imaging).

cases compared with SPECT and in 21% compared with CT. A more recent paper comparing $^{68}$Ga-DOTA-TATE PET/CT with SRS reported that in patients with negative or weakly positive findings on SRS, PET/CT documented 168 versus 28 lesions.[12] $^{68}$Ga-DOTA-peptides were also reported to influence the clinical management of patients with NET[13]: in a population of 90 cases with biopsy-proved NET, $^{68}$Ga-DOTA-NOC PET/CT findings affected either stage classification or therapy modifications in half the patients.

Moreover, $^{68}$Ga-DOTA-peptides PET/CT uptake correlates with SSR expression on NET cells,[14,15] and therefore provides an indirect measure of cells differentiation. Lesions with a high $^{68}$Ga-DOTA-peptide uptake have a higher differentiation grade and are therefore associated with a better prognosis[14] and are more likely to respond to treatment with either hot or cold somatostatin analogues. Semiquantitative and visual interpretation of the uptake of $^{68}$Ga-DOTA-peptides measured by PET/CT is currently used for guiding the quantity of radiation and the timing for targeted radionuclide therapy, using $^{177}$Lu or $^{90}$YDOTA-TOC. In this setting, $^{68}$Ga-DOTA-peptides PET/CT represents an indispensable procedure before planning target treatment with somatostatin analogues. However, considering the ligand/receptor mechanism of tracer uptake, $^{68}$Ga-DOTA-peptides do not represent the radiopharmaceuticals of choice to study the response to treatment, whereas metabolic tracers (eg, $^{18}$F-DOPA) are more suitable.

PET/CT with $^{68}$Ga-DOTA-peptides has also been successfully used for the detection of the unknown primary tumor site in patients with biopsy-proved secondary lesions[16,17] and negative physical examination, laboratory tests, and conventional imaging procedures (including chest radiograph, abdominal and pelvic CT, and mammography in women).

## COMPARISON OF $^{68}$GA-DOTA-PEPTIDES WITH METABOLIC TRACERS

Studies of direct comparison between $^{68}$Ga-DOTA-peptides imaging and $^{18}$F-DOPA are few and demonstrate the superiority of $^{68}$Ga-DOTA-peptides in well-differentiated forms of NET for the detection of the primary tumor and of secondary lesions.[15–17] These findings, in addition to $^{68}$Ga-DOTA-peptides easy and economic synthesis process and the possibility to study SSR expression before treatment, account for the increasing use of these compounds over $^{18}$F-DOPA in well-differentiated NET. On the contrary, $^{18}$F-DOPA may still offer advantages for the detection of tumors with a low or absent expression of SSR

(eg, medullary thyroid carcinoma, neuroblastoma) and to study disease at sites of known physiologic $^{68}$Ga-DOTA-peptides uptake (eg, adrenals).

Although generally considered inappropriate for the detection of NET lesions, because of slow glucose metabolism of well-differentiated forms, FDG may still prove valuable in case of low-grade tumors or in forms with variable or low SSR expression. Moreover, $^{18}$F-FDG may provide relevant prognostic information because the detection of highly metabolic lesions is associated with a worst outcome.[18,19]

## $^{68}$GA-DOTA-PEPTIDES PET/CT IMAGING PROTOCOL

The European Association of Nuclear Medicine recently published guidelines for $^{68}$Ga-DOTA-peptides PET/CT image acquisition and image interpretation.[9] $^{68}$Ga may be eluted from a commercially available $^{68}$Ge/$^{68}$Ga generator and the labeling of the DOTA-peptide with $^{68}$Ga is performed following standard procedures using semiautomated or fully automated systems. Either they are based on prepurification and concentration of the generator eluate using an anion-exchange[20,21] or cation-exchange technique,[22,23] or they use a fraction of the generator eluate directly for radiolabeling.[24,25] Radiolabeling is being performed using a suitable buffer at elevated temperature followed by chromatographic purification of the radiolabeling solution using a C-18 cartridge and an appropriate aseptic formulation. The method used ensures a level of $^{68}$Ga in the final preparation lower than 0.001% of the $^{68}$Ga radioactivity. Quality control protocols include tests for radionuclide purity; radiochemical purity (high-performance liquid chromatography, thin-layer chromatography); chemical purity (buffer, solvents); and sterility and endotoxin testing using validated methods.[9]

PET/CT imaging is performed (**Table 1**) after the intravenous administration of approximately 100 MBq (75–250 MBq) of the radiolabeled peptide ($^{68}$Ga-DOTA-NOC, DOTA-TOC, DOTA-TATE). Images are generally acquired after an uptake time of 60 minutes (45–90 minutes). $^{68}$Ga-DOTA-peptides physiologic uptake areas include the pituitary

| Table 1 | |
|---|---|
| **$^{68}$Ga-DOTA-peptides PET/CT imaging protocol** | |
| Patient preparation | None required |
| Dose (MBq) | 110 (75–250) |
| Uptake time (min) | 60 (45–90) |

<table>
<tr><td>

**Box 1**
**$^{68}$Ga-DOTA-peptides PET/CT pitfalls**

False-positives

    Accessory spleens

    Inflammation

    Lymphoma

    Head of the pancreas

False-negatives

    Small lesions size (<5 mm)

    Low/variable SSR expression

        Medullary thyroid cancer

        Neuroblastoma

        Pheocromocitoma

        Insulinoma

</td></tr>
</table>

gland; the spleen; the liver; the adrenal glands; the head of the pancreas; the thyroid (very mild uptake); and the urinary tract (kidneys and urinary bladder).

It is to be noted that no specific patient preparation is warranted before scanning. In particular, neither fasting nor discontinuation of somatostatin analogues treatment is required before imaging.[9] Patients are encouraged to void before image acquisition to reduce the background noise and the radiation dose to kidneys and bladder. Finally, the use of contrast media is not recommended for routine scanning.[26]

## PITFALLS IN IMAGE INTERPRETATION

False-positive reporting (**Box 1**) may derive from the presence of accessory spleens, inflammation, and lymphoma (caused by the presence of SSR on activated lymphocytes). Increased tracer uptake at the head of the pancreas is also a condition that can be associated with false-positive reporting. $^{68}$Ga-DOTA-peptide uptake in the esocrine pancreas (head) is a relatively frequent finding (DOTA-TOC, 67.8%[7]; DOTA-NOC, 31%[27]) not necessarily associated with the presence of disease.

False-negative findings (see **Box 1**) include small lesions dimension (<5 mm) and tumors with low or variable expression of SSR (eg, medullary thyroid carcinoma, neuroblastoma, insulinoma, pheocromocytoma).

## SUMMARY

$^{68}$Ga-DOTA-peptides currently represent the most promising tracers to study well-differentiated NET;

however, their use is limited to specialized centers in Europe as parts of clinical trials (**Box 2**). $^{68}$Ga-DOTA-peptides PET/CT are accurate for imaging NET lesions at the primary and metastatic sites (node, bone, liver, and unusual localizations). The advantages of their use over metabolic tracers ($^{18}$F-DOPA, $^{18}$F-FDG) are not only limited to a better overall detection rate but also to the fact that they provide data on SSR expression on target lesions, resulting a fundamental procedure before starting therapy with either hot or cold somatostatin analogues. From a technical point of view the easy and economic synthesis process of these compounds renders them suitable for use even in small centers without an on-site cyclotron.

The successful results obtained using $^{68}$Ga-DOTA-peptides PET/CT for NET imaging have raised questions regarding the current role of SRS. Certainly, SRS is still a valid tool to study NET. However, the possibility to use PET/CT with $^{68}$Ga-DOTA-peptides, when available, offers

<table>
<tr><td>

**Box 2**
**What the referring physician needs to know**

- $^{68}$Ga-DOTA-peptides (DOTA-TOC, DOTA-NOC, DOTA-TATE)

    Comparable diagnostic accuracy

    Overall sensitivity 90%–98%

    Overall specificity 92%–98%

    Uptake correlates with SSR expression

    Indications for NET imaging

        Staging/restaging

        Unknown primary tumor site detection

        Selection of patients for target therapy

        Detection of relapse/follow-up

- Advantages of the use of $^{68}$Ga-DOTA-peptides over metabolic tracers

    Higher detection rate (well-differentiated forms)

    Information on SSR expression on NET cells

    Easy and economic synthesis process

- Advantages of the use of $^{68}$Ga-DOTA-peptides PET/CT over SRS

    Higher spatial resolution

    Lower physiologic uptake in the liver and bowel

    Patient friendly (2 hours vs 4–24 hours)

    Better dosimetry

    Lower costs

</td></tr>
</table>

several advantages. In our opinion, the choice between the two imaging modalities should be performed taking into account local availability and expertise and the potential impact on patients' management. It is to be noted that the mere detection of a higher number of metastatic lesions by PET/CT compared with morphologic imaging or SRS is not always followed by a change in the therapeutic approach. On the contrary, the detection of unsuspected metastatic spread or local relapse, the identification of the site of the occult primary tumor, or the confirmation or exclusion of SSR on tumor cells are all conditions that can affect management. Therefore, if SRS is performed, PET/CT should be recommended only in cases in which the detection of a more extensive disease would change the therapeutic approach (eg, SRS-negative cases, cases in which SRS showed only the primary, equivocal SRS findings).

Finally, although a detailed analysis of the role of [18]F-FDG is beyond the scope of this article, it is worth mentioning that it may provide valuable information in NET forms characterized by a lower differentiation grade. Although it is well known that [18]F-FDG has a limited role in the assessment of well-differentiated forms, because of their slow glucose metabolic rate, it should also be reminded that NET may show variable degrees of differentiation between patients and in different lesions within the same patient. From a prognostic point of view, the detection of FDG-avid lesions is associated with a worse prognosis, reflecting the presence of lesions with a lower differentiation grade.

# REFERENCES

1. Krenning EP, Kwekkeboom DJ, Bakker WH, et al. Somatostatin receptor scintigraphy with [111In-DTPA-D-Phe1]-and [123I-Tyr3]-octreotide: the Rotterdam experience with more than 1000 patients. Eur J Nucl Med 1993;20:716–31.
2. Kowalski J, Henze M, Schuhmacher J, et al. Evaluation of positron emission tomography imaging using [68Ga]-DOTA-D-Phe1-Tyr3-octreotide in comparison to [111In]-DTPAOC SPECT. First results in patients with neuroendocrine tumors. Mol Imaging Biol 2003;5:42–8.
3. Buchmann I, Henze M, Engelbrecht S, et al. Comparison of 68Ga-DOTATOC PET and 111In-DTPAOC (Octreoscan) SPECT in patients with neuroendocrine tumours. Eur J Nucl Med Mol Imaging 2007;34(10):1617–26.
4. Antunes P, Ginj M, Zhang H, et al. Are radiogallium-labelled DOTA-conjugated somatostatin analogues superior to those labelled with other radiometals? Eur J Nucl Med Mol Imaging 2007;34(7):982–93.
5. Reubi JC. Peptide receptors as molecular targets for cancer diagnosis and therapy. Endocr Rev 2003;24(4):389–427.
6. Reubi JC, Waser B. Concomitant expression of several peptide receptors in neuroendocrine tumors: molecular basis for in vivo multireceptor tumour targeting. Eur J Nucl Med Mol Imaging 2003;30(5):781–93.
7. Gabriel M, Decristoforo C, Kendler D, et al. 68Ga-DOTA-Tyr3-octreotide PET in neuroendocrine tumors: comparison with somatostatin receptor scintigraphy and CT. J Nucl Med 2007;48(4):508–18.
8. Ambrosini V, Campana D, Tomassetti P, et al. 68Ga-labelled peptides for diagnosis of gastroentero-pancreatic NET. Eur J Nucl Med Mol Imaging 2012;39(Suppl 1):S52–60.
9. Virgolini I, Ambrosini V, Bomanji JB, et al. Procedure guidelines for PET/CT tumour imaging with 68Ga-DOTA-conjugated peptides: 68Ga-DOTA-TOC, 68Ga-DOTA-NOC, 68Ga-DOTA-TATE. Eur J Nucl Med Mol Imaging 2010;37(10):2004–10.
10. Poeppel TD, Binse I, Petersenn S, et al. 68Ga-DOTATOC versus 68Ga-DOTATATE PET/CT in functional imaging of neuroendocrine tumors. J Nucl Med 2011;52(12):1864–70.
11. Kabasakal L, Demirci E, Ocak M, et al. Comparison of 68Ga-DOTATATE and 68Ga-DOTANOC PET/CT imaging in the same patient group with neuroendocrine tumours. Eur J Nucl Med Mol Imaging 2012;39(8):1271–7.
12. Srirajaskanthan R, Kayani I, Quigley AM, et al. The role of 68Ga-DOTATATE PET in patients with neuroendocrine tumors and negative or equivocal findings on 111In-DTPA-octreotide scintigraphy. J Nucl Med 2010;51(6):875–82.
13. Ambrosini V, Campana D, Bodei L, et al. 68Ga-DOTANOC PET/CT clinical impact in patients with neuroendocrine tumors. J Nucl Med 2010;51(5):669–73.
14. Campana D, Ambrosini V, Pezzilli R, et al. Standardized uptake values of (68)Ga-DOTANOC PET: a promising prognostic tool in neuroendocrine tumors. J Nucl Med 2010;51(3):353–9.
15. Kaemmerer D, Peter L, Lupp A, et al. Molecular imaging with 68Ga-SSTR PET/CT and correlation to immunohistochemistry of somatostatin receptors in neuroendocrine tumours. Eur J Nucl Med Mol Imaging 2011;38(9):1659–68.
16. Prasad V, Ambrosini V, Hommann M, et al. Detection of unknown primary neuroendocrine tumours (CUP-NET) using (68)Ga-DOTA-NOC receptor PET/CT. Eur J Nucl Med Mol Imaging 2010;37(1):67–77.
17. Haug A, Auernhammer CJ, Wängler B, et al. Intraindividual comparison of 68Ga-DOTA-TATE and 18F-DOPA PET in patients with well-differentiated

metastatic neuroendocrine tumours. Eur J Nucl Med Mol Imaging 2009;36(5):765–70.

18. Ambrosini V, Tomassetti P, Castellucci P, et al. Comparison between 68Ga-DOTA-NOC and 18F-DOPA PET for the detection of gastro-entero-pancreatic and lung neuroendocrine tumours. Eur J Nucl Med Mol Imaging 2008;35(8):1431–8.

19. Koopmans KP, Neels ON, Kema IP, et al. Molecular imaging in neuroendocrine tumors: molecular uptake mechanisms and clinical results. Crit Rev Oncol Hematol 2009;71(3):199–213.

20. Velikyan I, Beyer GJ, Långström B. Microwave-supported preparation of 68Ga bioconjugates with high specific radioactivity. Bioconjug Chem 2004;15: 554–60.

21. Meyer GJ, Maecke H, Schuhmacher J, et al. 68Ga-labelled DOTA-derivatised peptide ligands. Eur J Nucl Med Mol Imaging 2004;31:1097–104.

22. Zhernosekov KP, Filosofov DV, Baum RP, et al. Processing of generator-produced 68Ga for medical application. J Nucl Med 2007;48:1741–8.

23. Di Pierro D, Rizzello A, Cicoria G, et al. Radiolabelling, quality control and radiochemical purity assessment of the octreotide analogue 68Ga DOTA NOC. Appl Radiat Isot 2008;66:1091–6.

24. Breeman WA, de Jong M, de Blois E, et al. Radiolabelling DOTA-peptides with 68Ga. Eur J Nucl Med Mol Imaging 2005;32:478–85.

25. Decristoforo C, Knopp R, von Guggenberg E, et al. A fully automated synthesis for the preparation of 68Ga-labelled peptides. Nucl Med Commun 2007; 28:870–5.

26. Mayerhoefer ME, Schuetz M, Magnaldi S, et al. Are contrast media required for (68)Ga-DOTA-TOC PET/CT in patients with neuroendocrine tumours of the abdomen? Eur Radiol 2012;22(4): 938–46.

27. Castellucci P, Pou Ucha J, Fuccio C, et al. Incidence of increased 68Ga-DOTANOC uptake in the pancreatic head in a large series of extrapancreatic NET patients studied with sequential PET/CT. J Nucl Med 2011;52(6):886–90.

# Role of $^{18}$F-Fluorodeoxyglucose PET in the Study of Neuroendocrine Tumors

Emmanouil Panagiotidis, MD, MSc,
Jamshed Bomanji, MBBS, PhD, FRCR, FRCP*

## KEYWORDS

- $^{18}$F-fluorodeoxyglucose (FDG) • Positron emission tomography (PET)
- Neuroendocrine tumors (NET) • Imaging • Prognosis

## KEY POINTS

- The most widely used PET radiopharmaceutical in daily clinical practice is $^{18}$F-fluorodeoxyglucose (FDG), an analogue of glucose with replacement of the oxygen in the C-2 position with fluorine-18.
- The evaluation of glycolytic metabolism by $^{18}$F-FDG is potentially useful in identifying high-risk patients with aggressive disease associated with a poor outcome.
- $^{18}$F-FDG may retain an important role in managing patients with neuroendocrine tumors owing to its high prognostic value and its higher sensitivity in delineating disease extent, especially in aggressive and high-grade tumors.
- With the advent of new combined modalities such as PET/MR imaging, more detailed information will become available on both morphologic and functional aspects, allowing better characterization of adrenal lesions and providing better delineation of the disease.
- The pivotal role of $^{18}$F-FDG in recurrent medullary thyroid cancer has been highlighted by several recent studies as the best second-line diagnostic method in patients with characteristics of aggressive disease, which include a high calcitonin (Ct) level of more than 1000 pg/mL, a short tumor Doubling times (Dts), an increased CEA level rather than increased Ct level and a high tumor proliferation index (Ki-67).
- Although the use of new somatostatin analogues labeled with 68-Gallium for PET has significantly increased the sensitivity of NET imaging compared with single photon emission computed tomography and $^{18}$F-FDG-PET, $^{18}$F-FDG may retain an important role in managing patients with NETs owing to its high prognostic value and its higher sensitivity in delineating disease extent, especially in aggressive and high-grade tumors.

## INTRODUCTION

Two of the most significant recent advances in medical imaging have been the introduction of Positron Emission Tomography (PET) and of the glucose analogue fluorodeoxyglucose (FDG) labeled with fluorine-18, which takes advantage of the process termed glycolysis in rapidly growing tumors.[1] Both now play an important role in cancer management in that they facilitate staging, evaluation of therapy response, restaging, and detection of recurrence.

Nuclear medicine imaging has been a powerful diagnostic tool for the management of patients with neuroendocrine tumors (NETs). NETs are

Disclosures: The authors have nothing to disclose.
Institute of Nuclear Medicine, University College London Hospitals NHS Trust, London, UK
* Corresponding author. Institute of Nuclear Medicine, University College Hospital, 235 Euston Road, London NW1 2BU, UK.
E-mail address: jamshed.bomanji@uclh.nhs.uk

PET Clin 9 (2014) 43–55
http://dx.doi.org/10.1016/j.cpet.2013.08.008
1556-8598/14/$ – see front matter © 2014 Elsevier Inc. All rights reserved.

epithelial neoplasms with neuroendocrine differentiation and include enterochromaffin cell tumors, sympathomedullary tumors such as neuroblastoma and pheochromocytoma, and medullary thyroid carcinoma (MTC). Because of the distinct pathophysiologic features of NETs, many radiopharmaceuticals have been investigated for use in PET imaging of these tumors, such as biogenic amine precursors (eg, fluorine-18 dihydroxyphenylalanine [$^{18}$F-DOPA]), somatostatin analogues (gallium-68 1,4,7,10-tetraazacyclododecane-1,4,7,10-tetra-acetic acid [DOTA]), hormone syntheses, and metabolic markers ($^{18}$F-FDG). The contribution of integrated functional and morphologic imaging modalities such as PET/computed tomography (CT) in overcoming the lack of anatomic tracer landmarking is significant.

It is well established that somatostatin analogues are the most useful and promising tracers for NET imaging, and they have the advantage of simultaneously providing dosimetry for peptide receptor radiotherapy. The published literature indicates that somatostatin analogues are highly sensitive in detecting less aggressive, well-differentiated NETs, whereas $^{18}$F-FDG is preferred for more aggressive, less-differentiated NETs. This article provides an update and overview of the role of $^{18}$F-FDG in the imaging of NETs.

## MECHANISM OF $^{18}$F-FDG UPTAKE

The most widely used PET radiopharmaceutical in daily clinical practice is $^{18}$F-FDG, an analogue of glucose with replacement of the oxygen in the C-2 position with fluorine-18. The half-life of $^{18}$F, 109.8 minutes, is sufficiently long for $^{18}$F-FDG to be transported to sites without a cyclotron. $^{18}$F-FDG is a tracer of energy substrate metabolism and is capable of depicting malignant tumors because they show increased glycolysis compared with normal tissues. In addition to malignant cells, $^{18}$F-FDG activity can be increased in activated macrophages, mainly in infection and inflammation.

$^{18}$F-FDG from the blood pool is transported into tumor cells by several membrane glucose transporter proteins (GLUT). Once intracellular, both glucose and $^{18}$F-FDG are phosphorylated by hexokinase as the first step in glycolysis. Once phosphorylated, glucose continues along the glycolytic pathway for energy production. However, FDG-6-phosphate does not undergo enzymatic reaction and remains effectively trapped intracellularly owing to its negative charge.

Tumor cells display an increased number of glucose transporters, particularly GLUT-1 and GLUT-3, as well as higher levels of hexokinase and isoforms type I and II. Glucose-6-phosphatase–mediated dephosphorylation of $^{18}$F-FDG occurs only slowly in most tumors, normal myocardium, and brain, and hence the uptake of this tracer is proportional to the glycolytic rate. However, tumors such as hepatocellular carcinoma and prostate carcinoma have higher glucose-6-phosphatase activity, resulting in low uptake.[2] Some tissues similarly have high glucose-6-phosphatase activity and show low uptake, including liver, kidney, intestine, and resting skeletal muscle.

Malignant cells are highly metabolically active, showing high mitotic rates and favoring the more inefficient anaerobic pathway; this adds to the already increased glucose demands, mainly caused by hypoxia, a common feature of tumor cells.[3] There are 2 main limitations of $^{18}$F-FDG. First, in addition to malignancies, lesions with a high concentration of inflammatory cells, such as neutrophils and activated macrophages, show increased $^{18}$F-FDG activity. Second, neoplasms with low glucose metabolism, such as well-differentiated NETs, show low $^{18}$F-FDG activity, reflecting the degree of tumor differentiation and their biologic behavior.

The use of $^{18}$F-FDG in NETs is controversial, probably owing to their low metabolic activity. Overall, the reported sensitivity is limited, but evidence is emerging that the presence of increased glucose in NETs highlights an increased propensity for invasion and metastasis, and overall poorer prognosis.

## NETS

NETs are a heterogeneous group of malignancies ranging from well-differentiated and slowly growing tumors to poorly differentiated and malignant neoplasms, which are less frequent and display aggressive behavior.[4] Neuroendocrine cells contain secretory granules having the capacity to produce biogenic amines and polypeptides.[5] Because they share the ability to accumulate and decarboxylate amine precursors such as L-DOPA and 5-hydroxytryptophan (5-HTP), neuroendocrine cells were classified as amine precursor uptake and decarboxylation cells.[5]

NETs may express hormonal activity similar to the endocrine cell from which they have originated, causing pronounced clinical symptoms. Functional NETs are characterized by a clinical or biochemical hormone excess, whereas nonfunctional NETs are devoid of clinically apparent hormonal activities despite hormone expression in the tumor being detected immunohistologically. Neuroendocrine cells also have the ability to express several different peptide receptors in high volumes, especially somatostatin receptors (SSRs), which are heptahelical G-protein–coupled glycoprotein transmembrane receptors.[6]

The older classification system for NETs, first proposed by Williams and Sandler[7] in 1963, was based on their embryologic site of origin. Foregut tumors, which account for nearly 25% of NETs, arise in the lung, thymus, stomach, or proximal duodenum. Midgut tumors, accounting for 50% of NETs, arise from the small intestine, the appendix (the most common site), or the proximal colon. Hindgut tumors, accounting for 15% of NETs, originate from the distal colon or rectum. Other sites of origin include gallbladder, kidney, liver, pancreas, thyroid, ovary, and testis.[8]

More recently, the World Health Organization (WHO) proposed a new classification system[9] in an attempt to clarify the classification of NETs and to standardize the system in a way that would enable clinicians to compare patients and predict outcomes. Under this system, NETs are classified into 3 broad categories:

1. Well-differentiated NETs, further subdivided into tumors that are benign and those with uncertain behavior (**Fig. 1**)
2. Well-differentiated (low-grade) neuroendocrine carcinomas with low-grade malignant behavior (**Fig. 2**)
3. Poorly differentiated (high-grade) NETs, which are the large cell neuroendocrine and small cell carcinomas (**Figs. 3 and 4**)

---

With regard to cellular grading, which reflects al aggressiveness, the grading system is based on 2 elements: (1) the rate of proliferation, which is defined by the number of mitoses (mitotic rate: number of mitoses per 10 high-power microscopic fields [HPFs]); and (2) the Ki-67 index, which is a proliferation index expressed as the percentage of tumor cells labeled by immunochemistry for this protein detected in nuclear fractions of proliferating cells in the $G_1$, $G_2$, and M phases of the cell cycle.

G1 grade: low proliferation index; Ki-67 less than or equal to 2% or 2 mitoses per HPF

G2 grade: moderate proliferation index; Ki-67 3% to 20% or 2 to 20 mitoses per HPF

G3 grade: high proliferation index; Ki-67 greater than 20% or greater than 20 mitoses per HPF

---

Imaging of NETs plays a crucial role in the diagnosis and management of the disease, largely owing to its ability to provide anatomic information for surgical planning. Important factors affecting the choice of method and combination of imaging modalities are the type of primary tumor, the presence or absence of hormonal activity (functionality), the presence of SSR, and the extent of disease. After histologic confirmation of disease, the initial diagnostic work-up and tumor staging form the basis for the decision to perform surgical resection or initiate medical therapy. Despite the small size of NETs compared with other malignancies, their impact on clinical status is significant owing to the release of hormones or biogenic amines. The small tumor size makes it difficult for conventional anatomic imaging to visualize the primary tumor or its metastases, given that these modalities are unable to depict specific endocrine features.

---

There are at least 4 radiopharmaceutical classes that address the different metabolic pathways or molecular properties of these tumors:

1. The glucose analogue $^{18}$F-FDG

2. Biogenic amine precursors such as $^{18}$F-dihydroxyphenylalaline or $^{11}$C-dihydroxyphenylalaline (DOPA), $^{18}$F-fluorodopamine, and $^{11}$C-HTP

3. Synthesis, storage, and hormone-releasing analogues and inhibitors such as $^{11}$C-hydroxyephedrine and the enzyme-inhibiting substrate $^{11}$C-metomidate

4. Peptide receptor ligands such as [$^{68}$Ga-DOTA$^0$-Tyr$^3$]octreotide ($^{68}$Ga-DOTATOC), [$^{68}$Ga-DOTA$^0$-Tyr$^3$]octreotate ($^{68}$Ga-DOTATATE), and [$^{68}$Ga-DOTA$^0$-1Nal$^3$]octreotide ($^{68}$Ga-DOTANOC), and $^{111}$In-diethylene triamine penta-acetic acid [$^{111}$In-DTPA$^0$]-octreotide-labeled somatostatin analogues.

---

### Enterochromaffin Cell Tumors

Enterochromaffin cells, first identified in 1897 by Kulchitsky, are a type of enteroendocrine cell occurring in the epithelia lining the lumen of the digestive tract and respiratory tract. The greek term entero refers to the gastrointestinal tract and chromaffin refers to the ability to stain with chromium or chrome salts, a common feature of serotonin-containing cells. The most common biologically active substance synthesized and secreted from enterochromaffin cells is serotonin, a vasoactive peptide whose release in the systemic circulation can cause the classic symptoms of carcinoid syndrome. Most enterochromaffin cell NETs are found within the gastrointestinal tract (55%) and bronchopulmonary system (30%).[10]

Because of the low metabolic activity and slow growth of NETs, $^{18}$F-FDG-PET/CT is usually reported to be of limited value in their management. In the early 1990s, Strauss and Conti[11] suggested

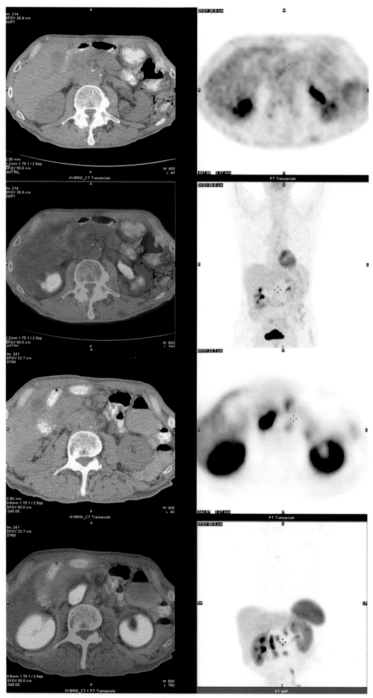

**Fig. 1.** Transaxial $^{68}$Ga-DOTATATE (*low panel*) and $^{18}$F-FDG-PET/CT (*upper panel*) images of a patient with small bowel carcinoid that was treated surgically. In follow-up studies there were $^{68}$Ga-DOTATATE–avid aortocaval, para-aortic, and mesenteric nodal deposits, but $^{18}$F-FDG negative. Histology revealed well-differentiated NET with KI-67 less than 2.

that despite these tumor characteristics, $^{18}$F-FDG might have a role in prognostic stratification in patients with NETs.

In 1998, in 7 patients with gastroenteropancreatic (GEP) tumors, Adams and colleagues[12] observed

an inverse relationship between $^{18}$F-FDG uptake and tumor differentiation, recognizing an association between increased glycolytic metabolism and high proliferative activity and poorly differentiated NETs. Pasquali and colleagues,[13] in the same

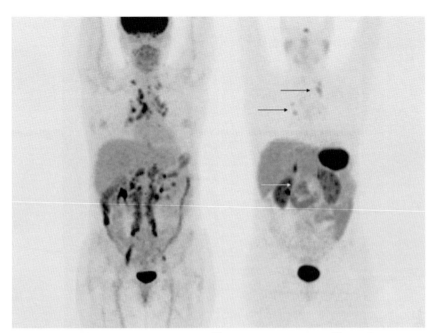

**Fig. 2.** Maximum intensity projection (MIP) images for 18F-FDG (*left panel*) and 68Ga-DOTATATE (*right panel*) in a female patient with a metastatic neuroendocrine carcinoma of unknown primary (Ki-67, 15%). There is positive uptake of 68Ga-DOTATATE (*arrows*) in lesions in the mediastinum and abdomen. However, the tumor shows more intense uptake of 18F-FDG, with many additional lesions not seen with 68Ga-DOTATATE.

year, found in 16 patients with carcinoids that 18F-FDG was positive at the primary tumor site in all patients with aggressive NETs. In contrast, in slow-growing NETs, 18F-FDG was negative in 7 patients and weakly positive in 1.

Belhocine and colleagues[14] compared 18F-FDG-PET with somatostatin receptor scintigraphy (SRS) using 111In-octreotide in a group of 17 patients with carcinoid tumors, most of which had a low Ki-67 proliferation index. They reported that 18F-FDG-PET had a low sensitivity of 57%, revealing 4 of 7 primary tumors, whereas SRS revealed 6 of the primary tumors. This finding led the investigators to conclude that 18F-FDG-PET should be reserved for patients with negative results on SRS.

Although the scintigraphic pattern of well-differentiated NETs with high uptake of somatostatin analogues and low glycolytic metabolism, and therefore low 18F-FDG activity, had been elucidated by previous studies, the relationship between tumor grade and scintigraphic pattern remained undocumented until Kayani and colleagues[15] compared the accuracy of 68Ga-DOTATATE and 18F-FDG based on Ki-67 and the mitotic index in 38 patients with a diagnosis of primary or recurrent GEP NETs. In this patient cohort, the activity of 68Ga-DOTATATE was higher in low-grade NETs (Ki-67 less than 2%) than in high-grade tumors (Ki-67 index more than 20%), which conversely showed significantly higher 18F-FDG

uptake. In patients with high-grade NETs, 77 of 79 detected lesions were positive with 18F-FDG, whereas only 5 were positive with 68Ga-DOTATATE. In those with low-grade NETs, 120 of 123 detected lesions were 68Ga-DOTATATE positive, whereas only 21 were positive with 18F-FDG. No lesion was depicted only by 68Ga-DOTATATE in patients with high-grade NETs or only by 18F-FDG in those with low-grade NETs.

The same author studied the diagnostic performance of the same radiotracers in 18 patients with pulmonary NETs, showing correlation with activity and tumor grade.[16] As with GEP NETs, a good association was observed between tumor grade and radiotracers' uptake. All 11 patients with typical carcinoids (low-grade tumors) showed high 68Ga-DOTATATE activity, whereas most showed low 18F-FDG uptake. In contrast, atypical and higher-grade tumors showed high 18F-FDG activity and low 68Ga-DOTATATE activity. Moreover, the specificity of 68Ga-DOTATATE was 100%, whereas 18F-FDG was false-positive in 3 cases. In this study, tumor type predicted the scintigraphic pattern but the Ki-67 index was determined in only 20% of patients, so no specific comparison of tumor grade was performed.

In another study, Binderup and colleagues[17] analyzed the diagnostic performance of 3 diagnostic modalities (111In-octreotide, 123I-metaiodobenzylguanidine [MIBG], and 18F-FDG-PET/CT)

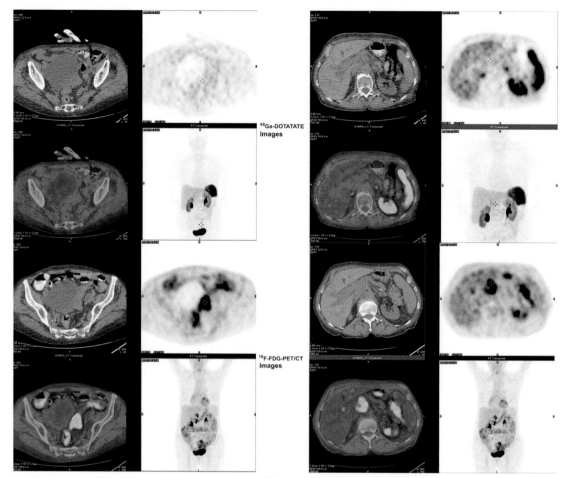

**Fig. 3.** Transaxial $^{68}$Ga-DOTATATE (*upper panel*) and $^{18}$F-FDG-PET/CT (*low panel*) images of a female patient with ovarian NET at staging. Primary mixed cystic and solid tumor is $^{68}$Ga-DOTATATE negative but $^{18}$F-FDG positive. There is also $^{18}$F-FDG–avid portal and paraortic nodal disease, which is negative in $^{68}$Ga-DOTATATE. Surgical removal of the tumor revealed poorly differentiated NET with KI-67 greater than 20.

in 96 patients with NETs according to the proliferation index. The overall sensitivity of SRS was significantly higher (89%) than that of $^{123}$I-MIBG (52%) and $^{18}$F-FDG (58%). There was a higher sensitivity of $^{18}$F-FDG (80%) in NETs with a proliferation index more than 2%, which increased to 92% for NETs with a proliferation index more than 15%. In contrast, the sensitivity of SRS was significantly higher for tumors with a proliferation index less than 15%.

Well-differentiated NETs are often low-grade lesions with a low Ki-67 index; the presence of a high Ki-67 index in this type of NET is important, not only because the proliferation index is a powerful prognostic tool but also because the choice of radiotracer for the functional examination is mainly based on tumor differentiation. Abgral and colleagues[18] recently compared the performance of $^{111}$In-octreotide, thoracoabdominopelvic CT, and $^{18}$F-FDG-PET/CT in a cohort of 18 consecutive

patients with aggressive well-differentiated NETs defined by a high Ki-67 index greater than or equal to 10. On a per-patient analysis, the sensitivity of SRS, CT, and $^{18}$F-FDG was 83%, 94%, and 100% respectively. On a per-lesion analysis, taking as a standard the highest number of distinct lesions visualized by at least 1 imaging method, the sensitivities of SRS, CT, and $^{18}$F-FDG were 43%, 77%, and 77% respectively. $^{18}$F-FDG was statistically significantly more sensitive than SRS for the diagnosis of lymph node involvement, with the best combination being $^{18}$F-FDG and CT, which allowed detection of 87% of lesions. The investigators proposed $^{18}$F-FDG as the radiotracer of first choice for staging metastatic well-differentiated NETs with a Ki-67 index of 10% or higher.

Based on this observation, there is a growing body of evidence that $^{18}$F-FDG is of prognostic value in patients with NETs. The first investigators to report an association between the intensity of

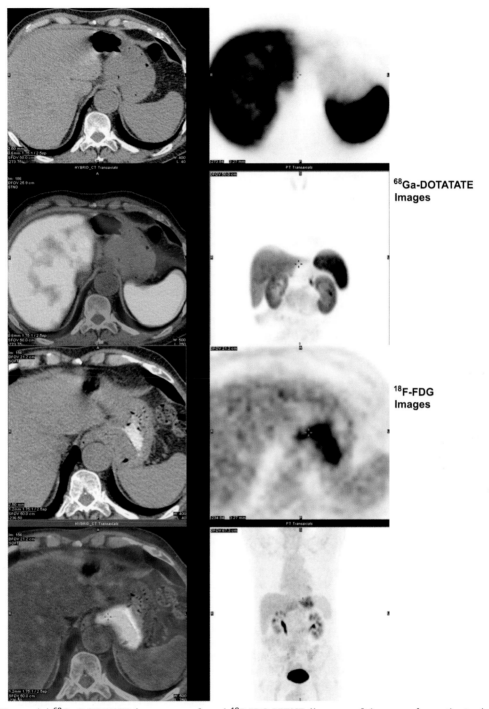

$^{68}$Ga-DOTATATE
Images

$^{18}$F-FDG
Images

**Fig. 4.** Transaxial $^{68}$Ga-DOTATATE (*upper panel*) and $^{18}$F-FDG-PET/CT (*low panel*) images of a patient who had subtotal gastrectomy for a high-grade neuroendocrine tumor of the stomach. There is recurrence of the tumor in proximity to the fundus of the stomach that is positive in $^{18}$F-FDG but negative in $^{68}$Ga-DOTATATE. Histology showed poorly differentiated NET with KI-67 greater than 20.

FDG activity and the survival of patients with NETs were Pasquali and colleagues[13] in 1998, supporting the evidence that an increased glycolytic rate indicates a worse prognosis. More recent studies have focused on the application of $^{18}$F-FDG-PET/CT in patients with aggressive NETs to determine prognostic metabolic features. Garin and colleagues[19] prospectively evaluated the prognostic value of $^{18}$F-FDG-PET/CT in 38 patients with metastatic NETs compared with $^{111}$In-octreotide and thoracoabdominal CT. On histology, 4 patients had high-grade NETs and 34 patients had low-grade NETs. Fourteen of 15 patients with positive PET had early progressive disease, whereas 21 of 23 patients with negative PET scans had stable disease. The overall positive and negative predictive values of $^{18}$F-FDG-PET/CT for the detection of disease progression within the first 6 months of follow-up were 93% and 91%, respectively. In the early prediction of rapidly progressive disease, $^{18}$F-FDG-PET/CT was more sensitive than pathologic differentiation and proliferative rate, and it was an independent predictive factor for progression-free survival.

A more recent study by Binderup and colleagues[20] examined a population of 98 patients with NETs in order to investigate the prognostic value of $^{18}$F-FDG in correlation with the proliferation index, liver metastases, and chromogranin A. During the 1-year follow-up, 14 patients died, of whom only 1 had a negative $^{18}$F-FDG-PET/CT examination; this shows that a positive $^{18}$F-FDG result is significantly associated with a higher risk of death in this group of patients. In this study, a maximum standardized uptake value ($SUV_{max}$) greater than 9 and a high Ki-67 index were significant predictors of overall survival, and the positive prognostic value of $^{18}$F-FDG-PET/CT for patient outcome was better than that of Ki-67 index, chromogranin A, and liver metastases, which are the traditional markers.

These results highlight the important role of $^{18}$F-FDG-PET/CT in the management of patients with NETs. The evaluation of glycolytic metabolism by the $^{18}$F-FDG-PET seems potentially useful in identifying high-risk patients with aggressive disease associated with a poor outcome. Although biopsy has the limitation that a tissue sample may not be representative of the whole tumor burden, $^{18}$F-FDG is also potentially of value in delineating not only the disease extent but also the preferred site for biopsy.

The management of patients with NETs depends primarily on the pathologic results (ie, low-grade vs high-grade malignancy). A strong association has recently been shown between high $^{18}$F-FDG uptake and worse patient outcome even in well-differentiated or low-grade tumors, with $^{18}$F-FDG-PET providing prognostic information independently of the mitotic rate. Although the use of new somatostatin analogues labeled with 68-Ga for PET has significantly increased the sensitivity of NET imaging compared with single-photon emission computed tomography and $^{18}$F-FDG-PET, $^{18}$F-FDG may retain an important role in managing patients with NETs owing to its high prognostic value and its higher sensitivity in delineating disease extent, especially in aggressive and high-grade tumors.

## Sympathomedullary Tumors

Sympathomedullary NETs are neoplasms arising from chromaffin tissue that develop into sympathetic and parasympathetic paraganglia throughout the body and synthesize catecholamines. Most of these tumors are located in the adrenal medulla and are called pheochromocytomas, but 10% arise from an extra-adrenal location near the celiac axis and are referred to as extra-adrenal pheochromocytomas or paragangliomas.

The incidence of pheochromocytoma is 2 to 8 per million persons per year. It presents in 0.1% to 1% of patients with hypertension and in approximately 5% of patients with an incidentally discovered adrenal mass.[21,22] The peak incidence occurs in the third and fifth decades of life, and the average age at diagnosis is 25 years in hereditary cases and 44 years in sporadic cases.[23] Of all the sympathomedullary NETs, 25% occur in the setting of a hereditary syndrome.[23] Major genetic syndromes that have been identified as carrying an increased risk of pheochromocytoma include multiple endocrine neoplasia (MEN) type 2A and 2B, von Hippel-Lindau disease, neurofibromatosis type I, and hereditary paraganglioma syndrome.

Once the biochemical diagnosis of pheochromocytoma or paraganglioma has been established from excess catecholamine secretion, imaging studies should be performed for the localization of the tumor in order to ascertain whether it is single or multiple, adrenal or ectopic, benign or malignant, and isolated or accompanied by other neoplasms in the context of familial syndrome.

The combination of anatomic imaging studies using CT or magnetic resonance (MR) imaging and functional imaging studies yields a sensitivity of nearly 100% for diagnosis of catecholamine-producing tumors.[24] Several studies have shown that $^{18}$F-FDG-PET/CT is a useful tool for assessment of chromaffin cell tumors, whether benign or malignant, with a sensitivity varying from 76% to 100%. Shulkin and colleagues[25] studied 29 patients with pheochromocytomas and reported a sensitivity of 76% (22/29). Most patients (7 of 12) with benign and nearly all patients (15 of 17) with malignant pheochromocytomas had $^{18}$F-FDG–avid tumors. $^{18}$F-FDG depicted disease in 4 patients who had negative $^{123}$I-MIBG imaging. However, in 9 patients (56%), $^{123}$I-MIBG had a superior target/background ratio, resulting in better delineation of the tumor.

Thirty patients who had succinate dehydrogenase subunit B (SDHB) germline mutation with metastatic pheochromocytoma/paraganglioma were studied by Timmers and colleagues[26] in order to evaluate the diagnostic performance of functional imaging modalities. Although not all the patients underwent all the modalities, sensitivity according to patient was 100% for [18]F-FDG, 88% for [18]F-dopamine (F-DA), 80% for [123]I-MIBG, and 81% for [111]In-pentetreotide (SRS). Moreover, 90% of regions that were false-negative on [123]I-MIBG or [18]F-DA were detected by [18]F-FDG. Therefore the investigators came to the conclusion that [18]F-FDG-PET/CT, with a sensitivity approaching 100%, is the preferred imaging modality for staging of SDH-related metastatic paraganglioma.

Taieb and colleagues[27] studied 9 patients with non-MEN2–related pheochromocytoma/paraganglioma, performing [18]F-FDG and [18]F-DOPA PET in all of them and [131]I-MIBG imaging in 8. Both PET tracers were superior to [131]I-MIBG, identifying additional tumor sites in 5 patients. [18]F-FDG was superior to [18]F-DOPA for the detection of adrenal and metastatic pheochromocytomas, whereas [18]F-DOPA and MIBG were more specific than [18]F-FDG. Compared with [18]F-DOPA, [18]F-FDG provided additional information in 3 cases of metastatic and abdominal paraganglioma but was inferior in cases of neck paraganglioma, leading the investigators to conclude that a combination of the two PET tracers is beneficial for preoperative work-up of patients with abdominal and malignant pheochromocytomas.

The same investigators evaluated [18]F-FDG-PET uptake in 28 patients with metastatic and nonmetastatic chromaffin-derived tumors, including 9 with genetically determined disease.[28] Twenty-six of the 28 (92%) patients showed significantly increased [18]F-FDG activity indicating disease. Furthermore, succinate dehydrogenase and von Hippel-Lindau–related tumors had significantly higher SUV$_{max}$ than neurofibromatosis and MEN type 2A syndrome–related tumors.

A retrospective analysis of the role of different modalities in the evaluation of bone involvement was performed by Zelinka and colleagues[29] in 71 subjects with metastatic paragangliomas and pheochromocytomas. The best overall sensitivity was shown by [18]F-DA (90%), followed by bone scintigraphy (82%), CT/MR imaging (78%), [18]F-FDG (76%), and [123/131]I-MIBG (71%). However, in subjects with the SDHB mutation, the best modality according to sensitivity was CT/MR imaging (96%), followed by bone scintigraphy (95%) and [18]F-FDG (92%). This finding led the author to the conclusion that [18]F-FDG-PET is highly recommended in this subgroup of patients.

In a small trial of 10 patients with 26 head and neck Succinate Dehydrogenase (SDHx)-related paragangliomas, King and colleagues[30] found that [18]F-FDG localized 20 of 26 lesions (77%) in 8 of 10 patients (80%), whereas [18]F-DOPA was positive in all of them. They suggested [18]F-DOPA as the first-line imaging agent for diagnosis and localization in this group of patients but, in the absence of [18]F-DOPA, [18]F-FDG should be used as an alternative.

In a recent study, Timmers and colleagues[31] investigated 216 patients for staging and characterization of chromaffin cell tumors. The sensitivity of [18]F-FDG (76.8%) was similar to that of [123]I-MIBG (75%) for nonmetastatic tumors but less than that of CT/MR imaging (95.7%). However, for metastatic disease the sensitivity of [18]F-FDG (82.51%) was greater than that of [123]I-MIBG (50%) and CT/MR imaging (74.4%), whereas for bone metastases it was further increased (93.7%). In conclusion, compared with [123]I-MIBG and CT/MR imaging, which have been considered gold standards for chromaffin cell imaging, [18]F-FDG performed better in depicting metastases, at the same time providing high specificity in patients with biochemically established disease.

In a prospective study, Takano and colleagues[32] found that both MR imaging with diffusion-weighted imaging (DWI) and [18]F-FDG showed all metastatic lesions in 11 patients with histologically confirmed chromaffin cell tumors, unlike [123]I-MIBG, which showed no metastatic lesions in 2 patients. Moreover, [123]I-MIBG failed to show many metastatic lesions that were detected by the other two modalities. MR imaging with DWI was advantageous in depicting lymph node and liver metastases, and showed a higher rate of detection of metastatic lesions compared with [123]I-MIBG or [18]F-FDG. However, [18]F-FDG was superior to MR imaging in showing mediastinal lymph node and lung metastases.

With the advent of new combined modalities such as PET/MR imaging, more detailed information will become available on both morphologic and functional aspects, allowing better characterization of adrenal lesions and providing better delineation of the disease.

## MTC

MTC is a rare, slow-growing NET originating from parafollicular C cells. It accounts for 5% to 8% of all thyroid cancers and has variable biological behavior and prognosis.[33] Management of MTC is difficult in both the sporadic (75%) and the familial form (25%), with an overall mean survival of 75% to 85% at 10 years.[33] Despite aggressive potentially curable treatment with total thyroidectomy and modified neck lymph node dissection, nearly 50% of the patients present with cervical or mediastinal lymph node recurrence and 10% to 20% have recurrence to the liver, lung, and bones.[34]

The therapeutic options are limited in those patients with metastatic disease, mainly because there is no tumor concentration of radioiodine and poor response to chemotherapy and radiation therapy.[35] The recent European Thyroid Association guidelines recommend surgery and other local treatment modalities (such as external beam radiation therapy, radiofrequency ablation, and chemoembolization) for the treatment of distant metastases in patients with low tumor burden (distant metastases limited to a single organ) and stable disease, whereas patients with symptoms, a significant tumor burden, and progressive disease should receive novel targeted systemic therapies.[36] Targeted therapy with vandetanib has shown promising results in the treatment of patients with metastatic and/or recurrent MTC.[37]

MTC secretes several neuroendocrine peptides, of which serum calcitonin (Ct) and the less specific carcinoembryonic antigen (CEA) are most frequently used as tumor markers for diagnosis, surveillance, and prognosis. However, conventional imaging is often negative in patients with a Ct concentration of less than 150 pg/mL, and identifies metastases in only about 40% of patients with biochemical evidence of recurrence.[36] In about one-third of patients with MTC lesions, CEA levels also may be increased. This finding has prognostic significance, because increased CEA levels are characteristic of advanced tumor forms with a tendency to dedifferentiation. Ct and CEA doubling times are efficient tools for assessing tumor progression and are useful prognostic factors for survival in patients with MTC; the probability of detecting metastases increases in patients with increasing tumor marker levels and shortening doubling times.[36] The recommended conventional imaging is extensive and comprises neck sonography for detection of cervical lymph node metastases; CT of the neck and thorax for lung, bone, and lymph node metastases; MR imaging for liver metastases; and bone scintigraphy. The success of [18]F-FDG-PET/CT in oncology imaging and the widespread use of PET/CT cameras in the last decade have provided an excellent alternative imaging modality for the management of MTC, especially in patients with negative conventional imaging.

A recent meta-analysis by Treglia and colleagues[38] on the performance of [18]F-FDG-PET or PET/CT in the detection of recurrent MTC covered 24 studies involving a total of 538 patients. The investigators showed a wide range of detection rates (24%–95%) on a per-patient analysis, the overall pooled detection rate being 59%. The investigators concluded that [18]F-FDG-PET/CT is not optimal in the surveillance of MTC because about 40% of suspected recurrences remain unidentified. False-negative results of [18]F-FDG could be related to small lesions or to the slow growth of NETs, both factors affecting its diagnostic accuracy. False-positive results usually occur because of inflammatory lesions.[37] The definition of false-negative and true-negative is ambiguous, because some investigators have considered patients with increased Ct concentrations and negative [18]F-FDG-PET/CT to have false-negative results, whereas others have considered them as true-negative.

In clinical practice, [18]F-FDG-PET/CT is usually performed in patients with biochemical evidence of MTC recurrence and no identified disease sites on conventional imaging or when calcitonin levels are out of proportion to the small volume of disease identified on conventional imaging. Moreover, the diagnostic ability of [18]F-FDG is greatly improved if patients with known lesions on conventional imaging are included in the study population, because functional abnormalities are usually detectable by [18]F-FDG when anatomic changes are already evident.[38]

Based on the literature findings, the diagnostic performance of [18]F-FDG in detecting recurrent MTC is significantly better in those patients with higher serum Ct/CEA levels and shorter Ct/CEA doubling times. This finding confirms the greater usefulness of [18]F-FDG in patients with more aggressive disease, which correlates with high glucose consumption and high [18]F-FDG uptake, compared with those with slowly progressive disease, which correlates with low glucose consumption and low [18]F-FDG uptake.[37]

In 28 patients with recurrent MTC, Ong and colleagues[39] found an overall sensitivity of 62%, which increased to 78% when Ct levels exceeded 1000 pg/mL. In contrast, all patients with a Ct of less than 500 pg/mL had negative [18]F-FDG, suggesting microscopic metastases or a low disease burden. Treglia and colleagues,[38] in a meta-analysis, found that the detection rate with [18]F-FDG-PET/CT (59%) increased to 69% if CEA was greater than or equal to 5 ng/mL, 75% if Ct was greater than or equal to 1000 ng/L, 76% if Ct doubling time was less than 12 months, and 91% if CEA doubling time was less than 24 months.

Comparative analyses of [18]F-DOPA and [18]F-FDG in the assessment of recurrent MTC have shown better results with $^{18}$F-DOPA in terms of sensitivity and specificity. This difference is mainly attributable to their different uptake mechanisms, reflecting different metabolic pathways in neuroendocrine cells: $^{18}$F-DOPA is a marker of amino acid decarboxylation, which is a feature of the neuroendocrine origin of MTC, and higher uptake is related to a higher degree of cell differentiation; in contrast, higher $^{18}$F-FDG uptake is related to high proliferative activity and poor differentiation.

In the study by Koopmans and colleagues,[40] 17 patients with recurrent MTC underwent both $^{18}$F-DOPA and $^{18}$F-FDG. The sensitivity of $^{18}$F-DOPA was higher than that of $^{18}$F-FDG on a per-patient analysis (62% vs 24%). Furthermore, there were discordant results in 7 of 17 (41%) patients, with $^{18}$F-DOPA PET/CT being positive and $^{18}$F-FDG-PET/CT negative for MTC recurrence in 6 patients. However, $^{18}$F-FDG was superior to $^{18}$F-DOPA in patients with a Ct doubling time of less than 12 months.

Kauhanen and colleagues[41] recently evaluated 19 patients with recurrent MTC using both methods, and reported $^{18}$F-DOPA to be superior to $^{18}$F-FDG (sensitivity in a per-patient analysis was 58% vs 53%). In most patients with MTC with occult disease, $^{18}$F-DOPA accurately detected metastases. In patients with unstable Ct levels, $^{18}$F-DOPA and $^{18}$F-FDG were complementary, whereas in patients with an unstable CEA doubling time $^{18}$F-FDG was more accurate. In a patient with a Ct of only 155 pg/mL, $^{18}$F-DOPA was the only method that accurately localized a metastasis in the neck/mediastinal region with a low Ki-67 proliferation index of 5%, indicating that $^{18}$F-DOPA PET/CT is of particular value for the detection of occult recurrent MTC characterized by a low proliferation index.

Based on the high-density expression of somatostatin receptors in NETs, $^{68}$Ga-somatostatin analogues have been used for MTC imaging, but on a limited scale. The only 2 retrospective studies of recurrent MTC have not indicated superiority of $^{68}$Ga-somatostatin analogues compared with $^{18}$F-FDG and/or $^{18}$F-DOPA.[42,43]

A recent multicentre study evaluated 18 cases of recurrent MTC using $^{18}$F-DOPA, $^{68}$Ga-somatostatin analogues, and $^{18}$F-FDG. The sensitivity of $^{18}$F-DOPA was higher than that of either $^{68}$Ga-somatostatin analogues or $^{18}$F-FDG in a per-patient analysis (72% vs 33.3% and 17%, respectively).[42] Lesion-based analysis showed $^{18}$F-FDG to be superior to $^{68}$Ga-somatostatin analogues, these modalities respectively detecting 20 and 14 of a total of 72 lesions and having a sensitivity of 28% and 20%. The investigator concluded that $^{18}$F-DOPA is the most useful radiotracer for detecting recurrent MTC, whereas $^{18}$F-FDG may complement $^{18}$F-DOPA in aggressive MTC.

In the second study, Conry and colleagues[43] found that, among 18 patients, $^{68}$Ga-DOTATATE PET/CT detected MTC recurrence in 13 patients (sensitivity 72%) and revealed 23 foci, whereas $^{18}$F-FDG-PET/CT detected recurrence in 14 patients (sensitivity 78%) and revealed 28 foci.

Although several recent studies have emphasized the pivotal role of $^{18}$F-FDG in recurrent MTC, conventional imaging is still recommended as the first-line approach. When conventional imaging fails to depict recurrent disease, the disease subtype should be the critical element in the selection of second-line imaging. $^{18}$F-FDG is the best second-line diagnostic method in patients with characteristics of aggressive disease, which include a high Ct level of more than 1000 pg/mL, a short tumor Dts, an increased CEA level rather than Ct increased level, and a high tumor proliferation index (Ki-67).

## REFERENCES

1. Wagner HN Jr. Clinical PET: its time has come. J Nucl Med 1991;32:561–4.
2. Torizuka T, Tamaki N, Inokuma T, et al. In vivo assessment of glucose metabolism in hepatocellular carcinoma with FDG-PET. J Nucl Med 1995;36:1811–7.
3. Minn H, Clavo AC, Wahl RL. Influence of hypoxia on tracer accumulation in squamous cell carcinoma: in vitro evaluation for PET imaging. Nucl Med Biol 1996;23:941–6.
4. Sundin A, Garske U, Orlesfors H. Nuclear imaging of neuroendocrine tumors. Best Pract Res Clin Endocrinol Metab 2007;21:69–85.
5. Pearse A. The APUD concept and hormone production. Clin Endocrinol Metab 1980;9:211–22.
6. Patel R, Kumar U, Lamb D, et al. Ligand binding to somatostatin receptors induces receptor-specific oligomer formation in live cells. Proc Natl Acad Sci U S A 2002;99:3294–9.
7. Williams ED, Sandler M. The classification of carcinoid tumours. Lancet 1963;1:238–9.
8. Modlin IM, Lye K, Kidd M. A 5-decade analysis of 13715 carcinoid tumours. Cancer 2003;97:934–59.
9. Solcia E, Kloppel G, Sobin LH. Histological typing of endocrine tumours. World Health Organization international histological classification of tumours. 2nd edition. Berlin: Springer; 2000.
10. Maggard MA, O'ConnelL J, Ko CY. Updated population-based review of carcinoid tumours. Ann Surg 2004;240:117–22.
11. Strauss LG, Conti PS. The application of PET in clinical oncology. J Nucl Med 1991;32:25.
12. Adams S, Baum R, Rink T, et al. Limited value of fluorine-18 fluorodeoxyglucose positron emission

tomography for the imaging of neuroendocrine tumours. Eur J Nucl Med 1998;25:79–83.

13. Pasquali C, Rubello D, Sperti C, et al. Neuroendocrine tumor imaging: can 18F-fluorodeoxyglucose positron emission tomography detect tumors with poor prognosis and aggressive behavior? World J Surg 1998;22:588–92.

14. Belhocine T, Foidart J, Rigo P, et al. Fluorodeoxyglucose positron emission tomography and somatostatin receptor scintigraphy for diagnosing and staging carcinoid tumours: correlation with the pathological indexed p53 and Ki-67. Nucl Med Commun 2002;23:727–34.

15. Kayani I, Bomanji JB, Groves A, et al. Functional imaging of neuroendocrine tumors with combined PET/CT using 68Ga-DOTATATE (DOTA-DPhe1, Tyr3-octreotate) and 18F-FDG. Cancer 2008;112:2447–55.

16. Kayani I, Conry B, Groves A, et al. A comparison of 68Ga-DOTATATE and 18F-FDG PET/CT in pulmonary neuroendocrine tumors. J Nucl Med 2009;50:1927–32.

17. Binderup T, Knigge U, Loft A, et al. Functional imaging of neuroendocrine tumors: a head-to-head comparison of somatostatin receptor scintigraphy, 123I-MIBG scintigraphy, and 18F-FDG PET. J Nucl Med 2010;51:704–12.

18. Abgral R, Leboulleux S, Déandreis D, et al. Performance of 18fluorodeoxyglucose-positron emission tomography and nuclear medicine imaging for GEPNET 183 somatostatin receptor scintigraphy for high Ki67 (≥10%) well-differentiated endocrine carcinoma staging. J Clin Endocrinol Metab 2011;96:665–71.

19. Garin E, Le Jeune F, Devillers A, et al. Predictive value of 18F-FDG PET and somatostatin receptor scintigraphy in patients with metastatic endocrine tumors. J Nucl Med 2009;50:858–64.

20. Binderup T, Knigge U, Loft A, et al. 18F-fluorodeoxyglucose positron emission tomography predicts survival of patients with neuroendocrine tumors. Clin Cancer Res 2010;16:978–85.

21. Omura M, Saito J, Yamaguchi K, et al. Prospective study on the prevalence of secondary hypertension among hypertensive patients visiting a general outpatient clinic in Japan. Hypertens Res 2004;27:193–202.

22. Young WF Jr. Management approaches to adrenal incidentalomas. A view from Rochester, Minnesota. Endocrinol Metab Clin North Am 2000;29:159–85.

23. Neumann H, Bausch B, McWhinney SR, et al. Germline mutations in nonsyndromic pheochromocytoma. N Engl J Med 2002;346:1459–66.

24. Ilias I, Pacak K. Current approaches and recommended algorithm for the diagnostic localisation of pheochromocytoma. J Clin Endocrinol Metab 2004;89:479–91.

25. Shulkin B, Thompson N, Shapiro B, et al. Pheochromocytomas: imaging with 2-[fluorine-18]fluoro-2-deoxy-D-glucose PET. Radiology 1999;212:35–41.

26. Timmers H, Kozupa A, Chen CC, et al. Superiority of fluorodeoxyglucose positron emission tomography to other functional imaging techniques in the evaluation of metastatic SDHB-associated pheochromocytoma and paragangioma. J Clin Oncol 2007;25:2262–9.

27. Taieb D, Tessonnier L, Sebag F, et al. The role of 18F-FDOPA and 18F-FDG PET in the management of malignant and multifocal phaeochromocytomas. Clin Endocrinol 2008;69:580–6.

28. Taieb D, Sebag F, Barlier A, et al. 18F-FDG avidity of pheochromocytomas and paragangliomas: a new molecular imaging signature? J Nucl Med 2009;50:711–7.

29. Zelinka T, Timmers HJ, Kozupa A, et al. Role of positron emission tomography and bone scintigraphy in the evaluation of bone involvement in metastatic pheochromocytoma and paraganglioma: specific implications for succinate dehydrogenase enzyme subunit B gene mutations. Endocr Relat Cancer 2008;15:311–23.

30. King K, Chen C, Alexopoulos D, et al. Functional imaging of SDHx-related head and neck paragangliomas: comparison of 18F-fluorodihydroxyphenylalanine, 18F-fluorodopamine, 18F-fluoro-2deoxy-D-glucose PET, 123I-metaiodobenzylguanidine scintigraphy and 111In-pentetreotide scintigraphy. J Clin Endocrinol Metab 2011;96:2779–85.

31. Timmers H, Chen C, Carrasquillo J, et al. Staging and functional characterization of pheochromocytoma and paragangliomas by 18F-fluorodeoxyglucose (18F-FDG) positron emission tomography. J Natl Cancer Inst 2012;104:700–8.

32. Takano A, Oriuchi N, Tsushima Y, et al. Detection of metastatic lesions from malignant pheochromocytoma and paragangliomas with diffusion-weighted magnetic resonance imaging: comparison with 18F-FDG positron emission tomography and 123I-MIBG scintigraphy. Ann Nucl Med 2008;22:395–401.

33. Pitt S, Moley F. Medullary, anaplastic, and metastatic cancers of the thyroid. Semin Oncol 2010;37(6):567–79.

34. Roman S, Mehta P, Sosa JA. Medullary thyroid cancer: early detection and novel treatments. Curr Opin Oncol 2009;21:5–10.

35. Wu LS, Roman SA, Sosa JA. Medullary thyroid cancer: an update of new guidelines and recent developments. Curr Opin Oncol 2011;23:22–7.

36. Schlumberger M, Bastholt L, Dralle H, et al. 2012 European Thyroid Association guidelines for metastatic medullary thyroid cancer. Eur Thyroid J 2012;1:5–14.

37. Wells S, Robinson B, Gagel R, et al. Vandetanib in patients with locally advanced or metastatic

medullary thyroid cancer: a randomized, double-blind phase III trial. J Clin Oncol 2012;30:134–41.

38. Treglia G, Villani MF, Giordano A, et al. Detection rate of recurrent medullary thyroid carcinoma using fluorine-18 fluorodeoxyglucose positron emission tomography: a meta-analysis. Endocrine 2012;42:535–45.

39. Ong S, Schoder H, Patel G, et al. Diagnostic accuracy of 18F-FDG PET in restaging patients with medullary thyroid carcinoma and elevated calcitonin levels. J Nucl Med 2007;48:501–7.

40. Koopmans KP, de Groot JW, Plukker JT, et al. 18F-dihydroxyphenylalanine PET in patients with biochemical evidence of medullary thyroid cancer: relation to tumor differentiation. J Nucl Med 2008;49:524–31.

41. Kauhanen S, Schalin-Jäntti C, Seppänen M, et al. Complementary roles of 18F-DOPA PET/CT and 18F-FDG PET/CT in medullary thyroid cancer. J Nucl Med 2011;52:1855–63.

42. Treglia G, Castaldi P, Villani MF, et al. Comparison of 18FDOPA, 18F-FDG and 68Ga-somatostatin analogue PET/CT in patients with recurrent medullary thyroid carcinoma. Eur J Nucl Med Mol Imaging 2012;39:569–80.

43. Conry BG, Papathanasiou ND, Prakash V, et al. Comparison of (68)Ga-DOTATATE and (18)F-fluorodeoxyglucose PET/CT in the detection of recurrent medullary thyroid carcinoma. Eur J Nucl Med Mol Imaging 2010;37:49–57.

# Other PET Tracers for Neuroendocrine Tumors

Klaas Pieter Koopmans, MD, PhD[a],*,
Andor W.J.M. Glaudemans, MD[b]

## KEYWORDS

- [11]C-5-HTP PET • [124]I-MIBG • Neuroendocrine tumor • Pancreatic islet cell tumor

## KEY POINTS

- [124]I-MIBG has superior resolution compared with [123]I-MIBG.
- [124]I-MIBG may potentially be a good tracer for neuroblastoma and pheochromocytoma.
- [124]I-MIBG is suitable for pre-[131]I-MIBG treatment dosimetry.
- [11]C-5-HTP has the highest detection of pancreatic islet cell tumors and metastases when compared with CT, [18]F-FDOPA, and SRS imaging.
- [11]C-5-HTP also has a high detection rate for carcinoids.

## INTRODUCTION

Gastro-enteropancreatic (GEP) neuroendocrine tumors (NETs) arise in the pancreas and gastrointestinal system (**Table 1**). These tumors are derived from neuroendocrine cells.

Well-differentiated GEP NETs generally have a low glucose metabolism, opposed to many other malignancies.[1,2] This low glucose metabolism of well-differentiated GEP NETs yields a limited value of [18]F-fluorodexyglucose ([18]F-FDG) PET scanning for the primary staging of these patients. Because primary tumors of GEP NETs can be very small in size and generally show only moderately increased glucose uptake, even in the metastases, [18]F-FDG PET may result in false negative findings. Therefore, as a staging tool, [18]F-FDG does not seem to have a place in the general GEP NET patient population.[1,3–5] This low FDG PET sensitivity for GEP NET, combined with the NETs-specific hormone production and receptor expression, has led to the development of more NET-specific tracers, of which [124]I-metaiodobenzylguanidine (MIBG) and β-[[11]C]-5-hydroxy-L-tryptophan ([11]C-5-HTP) are discussed here.

GEP NETs often show increased synthesis and secretion of hormones and neurotransmitters. Nontumorous neuroendocrine cells regulate a variety of body functions through paracrine stimulation with a large variety of hormones and neurotransmitters. Serotonin, catecholamine, and histamine are examples of compounds that share specific steps in their biosynthesis and storage, such as decarboxylation before storage in granules.[6] In GEP NETs, the catecholamine and serotonin biosynthetic pathways are up-regulated especially. Increased biosynthesis of these specific amines in GEP NETs enables imaging with specific amine precursors. In this article imaging of cells that show increased production of catecholamine and/or serotonin are discussed for GEP NETs encompassing NETs from foregut (bronchus, lung, thymus, stomach, pancreas, and proximal duodenum), mid gut (from the distal half of the second part of the duodenum to the proximal two-thirds of the transverse colon), and hindgut (descending colon, sigmoid and rectum) origin.

Disclosures: The authors have nothing to disclose.
[a] Department of Radiology and Nuclear Medicine, Martini Hospital Groningen, Van Swietenplein 1, Groningen 9728 NT, The Netherlands; [b] Department of Nuclear Medicine and Molecular Imaging, University Medical Center Groningen, University of Groningen, Groningen, The Netherlands
* Corresponding author.
E-mail address: k.koopmans@mzh.nl

PET Clin 9 (2014) 57–62
http://dx.doi.org/10.1016/j.cpet.2013.08.009

**Table 1**
**Imaging protocols**

|  | [124]I-MIBG[10,23] | [11]C-5-HTP[17] |
|---|---|---|
| Patient preparation | — | 2-h fasting |
| Tracer dose | 50 MBq | 200 MBq or 1.5 MBq/kg |
| Other? | Thyroid blocking 24 h before injection | Carbidopa 2.5 mg/kg 1 h before injection |
| Waiting time before scan | 48 h | 10 min |

## MIBG IMAGING THE CATECHOLAMINE PATHWAY

The precise uptake and retention mechanism in NETs for MIBG have not been clarified, but the noradrenalin transporter seems to play an important role for MIBG uptake (**Figs. 1–3**). Reports indicate that MIBG acts as an intracellular substrate for the vesicular monoamine transporters VMAT1 and VMAT2.[7,8] These transporters are located on the membrane of secretory vesicles of neuroendocrine cells. From the available data, it seems likely that once MIBG has passed the cell membrane, the VMAT transporters transport MIBG into secretory chromaffin granules.[9]

MIBG has traditionally been labeled with [123]I and [131]I, but lately reports have become available whereby [124]I MIBG has been used clinically for the detection of pheochromocytomas.[10] In preclinical and clinical settings, its potential usefulness in patients with neuroblastomas was evaluated.[11,12] [124]I-MIBG is a PET tracer, which theoretically and practically yields a better image quality, due to the superior resolution of the PET camera system when compared with conventional gamma

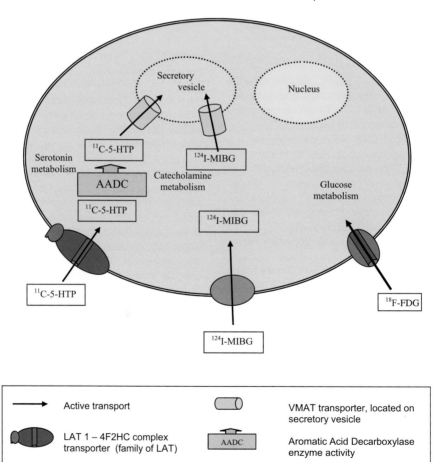

**Fig. 1.** A schematic overview is presented of uptake mechanisms of the tracers described in this article.

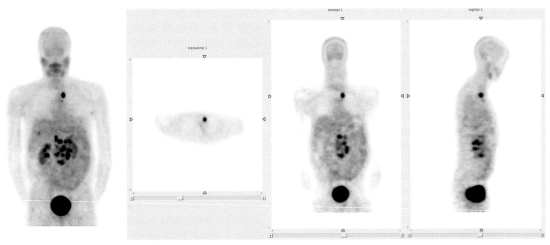

**Fig. 2.** $^{11}$C-5-HTP PET/CT. Images of a 54-year-old man with a carcinoid. $^{11}$C-5-HTP PET with carbidopa pretreatment. Physiologic excretion of $^{11}$C-5-HTP metabolites is via kidneys with physiologic activity in the ureters and urinary bladder. Metastases are visible in the mediastinum, liver, and intra-abdominal area.

camera imaging. With an estimated effective dose, conform International Commission on Radiological Protection 103, of 3.75 mSv/MBq for children to 0.24 mSv/MBq for male adults, it has a lower radiation burden than $^{124}$I sodium iodine (NaI), used for imaging thyroid carcinoma.[13] $^{123}$I-MIBG scintigraphy and (after therapy) $^{131}$I-MIBG scintigraphy have become the imaging method of choice for neuroblastoma and pheochromocytomas and most likely $^{124}$I-MIBG will follow. In children with neuroblastoma especially, $^{124}$I-MIBG may become an important tool in staging disease and performing dosimetry before therapy.[12]

However, for GEP NETs MIBG scintigraphy and likely also $^{124}$I-MIBG PET scanning has a lower

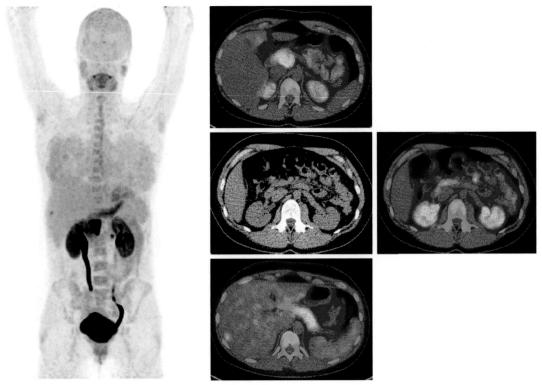

**Fig. 3.** $^{11}$C-5-HTP PET/CT of a female patient with an insulinoma in the head of the pancreas, a lymph node metastasis in the mesentery, and a small metastasis in the liver.

sensitivity for the detection of other NETs, such as carcinoids (averaging 50%).[14]

## β-[¹¹C]-5-HTP IMAGING THE SEROTONIN PATHWAY

Serotonin is a monoamine neurotransmitter, present in blood platelets and in the intestinal wall where it regulates contractions. In the brain, serotonin acts as a neurotransmitter.

The serotonin pathway shares the large amino acid transporter (LAT) and vesicular monoamine transporter (VMAT) transporter systems with the catecholamine pathway. The enzyme AADC plays a key role in the final step for the synthesis of serotonin as a functional hormone.

In the serotonin pathway the amino acid tryptophan and the intermediate product 5-HTP are precursors for serotonin after uptake via the LAT system. The regulation of this uptake mechanism is still unclear. After decarboxylation via the enzyme AADC, serotonin is taken up via VMAT transporters into storage vesicles from which it can be released extracellularly (see **Fig. 1**). Serotonin is eventually metabolized to 5-hydroxyindole acetic acid (5-HIAA), which is secreted in the urine.

In many NETs the serotonin pathway is overactive. Therefore, the development of a PET tracer for NETs exploiting this pathway is of invaluable importance.[6] The serotonin pathway has proven to be a difficult target for tracer development, because until now only a carbon-11-labeled tracer has been developed for the serotonin pathway, ¹¹C-5-HTP. The tracer ¹¹C-5-HTP was developed in Uppsala, Sweden, during the 1980s. The synthesis of this tracer is difficult, because it demands an on-site cyclotron for the production of a large amount of ¹¹C isotope (with a half-life of only 20 minutes), followed by a long, 2-multienzyme-step, synthesis.[15,16] Only a few centers worldwide are able to produce ¹¹C-5-HTP. However, in experienced hands quantities up to 1000 MBq can be reliably synthesized for (clinical) use. Image interpretation is mostly easy due to high tumor tracer uptake and low background uptake in normal tissues. Although difficult to produce, this tracer has proven itself clinically for the detection of GEP NETs.[17]

In 1993 the first results with this tracer were published.[18] Nowadays, ¹¹C-5-HTP PET scanning is typically performed 10 to 20 minutes after injection of ¹¹C-5-HTP with carbidopa pretreatment, 2 mg/kg body weight, or with a fixed dose of 200 mg, 1.5 hours before injection. No adverse reactions after the intravenous injection of ¹¹C-5-HTP have thus far been reported.

In contrast to ¹⁸F-FDOPA PET scans, carbidopa pretreatment is essential for a good image quality with ¹¹C-5-HTP PET. Carbidopa pretreatment reduces urinary excretion of ¹¹C-5-HTP, thereby reducing reconstruction artifacts in the area of the kidneys, ureters, and urinary bladder. It is hypothesized that carbidopa decreases the peripheral decarboxylation of ¹¹C-5-HTP to ¹¹C-5-HT (serotonin) and the subsequent urinary excretion of ¹¹C-serotonin metabolites. This reduction in peripheral decarboxylation and excretion can lead to a higher availability of tracer for tumor uptake. This effect has been tested in patients with mid-gut carcinoids, who were scanned with and without carbidopa pretreatment 1 hour before injection of ¹¹C-5-HTP. In this study, oral carbidopa pretreatment significantly reduced urinary radioactivity concentration from a mean standardized uptake value (SUV) of the pelvis of 155 ± 195 to 39 ± 14 SD, which led to an improved image quality in that area. Interestingly, tumor uptake of ¹¹C-5-HTP significantly increased, from 11 ± 3 to 14 ± 3 SD, and pancreatic uptake decreased slightly, to a SUV of 4.4 ± 0.8 SD. In liver tissue a small increase of ¹¹C-5-HTP uptake after oral carbidopa administration was found, now reaching an SUV of 3.6 ± 0.8 (before). A possible explanation for this increased ¹¹C-HTP liver uptake has not been described yet.[19]

Only a few studies with a reasonable number of patients with GEP NETs have thus far been published. In 1998, Orlefors and colleagues[20] published the first study with ¹¹C-5-HTP PET. In this study 18 patients with histopathologically verified NETs were included: midgut (n = 14), foregut (n = 1), hindgut carcinoid (n = 1), and endocrine pancreatic tumors (n = 2). ¹¹C-5-HTP PET without oral carbidopa pretreatment was compared with computed tomography (CT). All 18 patients showed increased ¹¹C-5-HTP uptake in tumor tissue. One patient with a hindgut carcinoid and one patient with a nonfunctioning endocrine pancreatic tumor with normal urinary 5-HIAA levels, suggesting a normal activity of the serotonin pathway, also showed increased tumor uptake. In this study, ¹¹C-5-HTP PET detected more tumor lesions than CT in 10 patients and was equal in 5 patients (4 mid-gut, 1 foregut), with missing data in 3 patients with mid-gut NET. In the 10 patients that were on treatment with interferon-α ± octreotide, or somatostatin analogue only, a close correlation between the changes in ¹¹C-5-HTP transport rate constant in the tumors and urinary 5-HIAA was noted. It was therefore suggested that ¹¹C-5-HTP PET may serve as a means to monitor therapy, although it is still unknown whether these PET findings under medication relate to changes in tumor metabolism or in changes in amine processing.[20]

In 2005, Orlefors and colleagues published another report in which 38 patients with a variety of NETs, consisting of mid-gut carcinoids (n = 13), lung carcinoids (n = 7), nonfunctioning endocrine pancreatic tumors (n = 5), and other NETs (n = 13), were evaluated with [11]C-5-HTP PET. In this study, whole-body [11]C-5-HTP PET imaging with oral carbidopa pretreatment was compared with both CT and somatostatin receptor scintigraphy (SRS). With whole-body [11]C-5-HTP PET scanning, tumor lesions in 36 of 38 (95%) patients were detected. In 84% of these patients SRS was abnormal, whereas CT was abnormal in 79%. More lesions were detected with [11]C-5-HTP PET in 22 of 38 (58%) patients compared with SRS and CT, whereas the imaging modalities showed equal numbers of lesions in 13 of 38 patients (34%). In 3 patients SRS or CT showed more lesions than [11]C-5-HTP PET. Patients with a nonfunctioning endocrine pancreatic tumor, and a pancreatic carcinoma with some endocrine differentiation on immunohistochemistry, did not show [11]C-5-HTP tumor uptake. In a patient with metastasized thymus carcinoma [11]C-5-HTP PET and SRS only showed the primary tumor, whereas CT scan also detected metastases. From these patients it was speculated that in the case of high proliferation rate and dedifferentiation of NETs, [18]F-FDG PET is probably the imaging modality of choice. In the 17 patients who had their primary tumor still in situ, [11]C-5-HTP PET was positive in 16, compared with SRS in 9, and CT in 8 patients. Surgically verified lesions as small as 6 mm could be detected with [11]C-5-HTP PET. The main conclusion of this study was that PET imaging with [11]C-5-HTP can be universally applied in NETs, also in patients without elevated 5-HIAA excretion in urine, as long as the tumor is not highly proliferating and/or dedifferentiating.[21,22]

In another study of 24 patients with carcinoid tumors and 23 patients with pancreatic islet cell tumors, [11]C-5-HTP PET was compared with conventional imaging with CT and SRS and a [18]F-FDOPA PET scan.[17] Whole-body PET images with carbidopa pretreatment were recorded 10 minutes after intravenous injection of [11]C-5-HTP, or 60 minutes after intravenous administration of [18]F-FDOPA. The PET findings were compared, per patient and per lesion, with a composite reference standard derived from all available imaging data along with clinical and cytologic/histologic information. Results indicated that indeed [11]C-5-HTP PET can be seen as a universal imaging agent for carcinoid and pancreatic islet cell tumor patients. In this series, [11]C-5-HTP PET was the only imaging modality positive in all patients (100% sensitivity). In islet cell tumor patients especially, more tumor-positive patients and lesions were found with [11]C-5-HTP (100% and 67%) compared with [18]F-FDOPA (89% and 41%), SRS (78% and 46%), and CT (87% and 68%). However, in carcinoid patients the per-lesion analysis showed that [18]F-FDOPA PET outperformed all other imaging techniques, including [11]C-5-HTP PET. Adding CT to both imaging techniques resulted in a further improvement in sensitivity in a per-lesion analysis, because both types of imaging techniques were complementary to each other. Therefore, for pancreatic islet cell patients [11]C-5-HTP PET/CT was considered the optimal imaging technique, whereas for carcinoid patients, [18]F-FDOPA PET/CT was considered the optimal imaging technique. Furthermore, it was stated that in carcinoid patients SRS scanning can be omitted without missing any lesions. In patients with islet cell tumors, SRS performed better than both PET techniques in a minority of patients (8%), and therefore remains of additional value.

Due to the difficult synthesis of [11]C-5-HTP, only a few centers worldwide are able to perform [11]C-5-HTP PET scanning. Therefore, assessing the place of [11]C-5-HTP PET in staging and monitoring disease and disease progression in GEP NETs is very important. A direct comparison between [11]C-5-HTP, [18]F-FDOPA, and the recently developed [68]Ga-labeled somatostatin analogues for PET imaging in various subtypes of NETs is warranted. It would also be highly beneficial when a serotonin analogue with a PET isotope with a longer half life, such as [18]Fluor, would become available. This way, the understanding of the role of serotonin PET analogues in the imaging of GEP NETs could be improved more easily.

## SUMMARY

[11]C-5-HTP PET is, according to the data available, an excellent functional imaging technique for evaluating patients with pancreatic islet cell tumors and, although with a slightly lesser sensitivity, also for carcinoids. However, it remains to be determined what the place is of [11]C-5-HTP PET in the workup of patients with a suspicion of GEP NET tumor. The major drawback of [11]C-5-HTP PET is the difficult synthesis and limited availability. The development of a [18]F-labeled serotonin precursor that performs at

least equal to the [11]C-5-HTP tracer would be very helpful. Although promising, at this time only case reports on the use of [124]I-MIBG in patients with GEP NETs are available. However, [124]I-MIBG is expected to be of great value in patients with neuroblastoma and pheochromocytoma.

## REFERENCES

1. Adams S, Baum R, Rink T, et al. Limited value of fluorine-18 fluorodeoxyglucose positron emission tomography for the imaging of neuroendocrine tumours. Eur J Nucl Med 1998;25(1):79–83.
2. Belhocine T, Foidart J, Rigo P, et al. Fluorodeoxyglucose positron emission tomography and somatostatin receptor scintigraphy for diagnosing and staging carcinoid tumours: correlations with the pathological indexes p53 and Ki-67. Nucl Med Commun 2002;23(8):727–34.
3. Pasquali C, Rubello D, Sperti C, et al. Neuroendocrine tumor imaging: can 18F-fluorodeoxyglucose positron emission tomography detect tumors with poor prognosis and aggressive behavior? World J Surg 1998;22(6):588–92.
4. Garin E, Le Jeune F, Devillers A, et al. Predictive value of 18F-FDG PET and somatostatin receptor scintigraphy in patients with metastatic endocrine tumors. J Nucl Med 2009;50(6):858–64.
5. Fiebrich HB, Brouwers AH, Koopmans KP, et al. Combining 6-fluoro-[18F]l-dihydroxyphenylalanine and [18F]fluoro-2-deoxy-d-glucose positron emission tomography for distinction of non-carcinoid malignancies in carcinoid patients. Eur J Cancer 2009;45(13):2312–5.
6. Jager PL, Chirakal R, Marriott CJ, et al. 6-L-18F-fluorodihydroxyphenylalanine PET in neuroendocrine tumors: basic aspects and emerging clinical applications. J Nucl Med 2008;49(4):573–86.
7. Kolby L, Bernhardt P, Levin-Jakobsen AM, et al. Uptake of meta-iodobenzylguanidine in neuroendocrine tumours is mediated by vesicular monoamine transporters. Br J Cancer 2003;89(7):1383–8.
8. Altmann A, Kissel M, Zitzmann S, et al. Increased MIBG uptake after transfer of the human norepinephrine transporter gene in rat hepatoma. J Nucl Med 2003;44(6):973–80.
9. Furuta N, Kiyota H, Yoshigoe F, et al. Diagnosis of pheochromocytoma using [123I]-compared with [131I]-metaiodobenzylguanidine scintigraphy. Int J Urol 1999;6(3):119–24.
10. Hartung-Knemeyer V, Rosenbaum-Krumme S, Buchbender C, et al. Malignant pheochromocytoma imaging with [124I]mIBG PET/MR. J Clin Endocrinol Metab 2012;97(11):3833–4.
11. Charron M. Contemporary approach to diagnosis and treatment of neuroblastoma. Q J Nucl Med Mol Imaging 2013;57(1):40–52.
12. Seo Y, Gustafson WC, Dannoon SF, et al. Tumor dosimetry using [124I]m-iodobenzylguanidine microPET/CT for [131I]m-iodobenzylguanidine treatment of neuroblastoma in a murine xenograft model. Mol Imaging Biol 2012;14(6):735–42.
13. Lee CL, Wahnishe H, Sayre GA, et al. Radiation dose estimation using preclinical imaging with 124I-metaiodobenzylguanidine (MIBG) PET. Med Phys 2010;37(9):4861–7.
14. Koopmans KP, Neels ON, Kema IP, et al. Molecular imaging in neuroendocrine tumors: molecular uptake mechanisms and clinical results. Crit Rev Oncol Hematol 2009;71(3):199–213.
15. Bjurling P, Watanabe Y, Tokushige M, et al. Syntheses of β-11C-labelled L-tryptophan and 5-hydroxy-L-tryptophan using a multi-enzymatic reaction route. J Chem Soc Perkin 1 1989;1(7):1331–4.
16. Neels OC, Jager PL, Koopmans KP, et al. Development of a reliable remote-controlled synthesis of β-[11C]-5-hydroxy-L-tryptophan on a Zymark robotic system. J Labelled Comp Rad 2006;49:889–95.
17. Koopmans KP, Neels OC, Kema IP, et al. Improved staging of patients with carcinoid and islet cell tumors with 18F-dihydroxy-phenyl-alanine and 11C-5-hydroxy-tryptophan positron emission tomography. J Clin Oncol 2008;26(9):1489–95.
18. Eriksson B, Bergstrom M, Lilja A, et al. Positron emission tomography (PET) in neuroendocrine gastrointestinal tumors. Acta Oncol 1993;32(2):189–96.
19. Orlefors H, Sundin A, Lu L, et al. Carbidopa pretreatment improves image interpretation and visualisation of carcinoid tumours with 11C-5-hydroxytryptophan positron emission tomography. Eur J Nucl Med Mol Imaging 2006;33(1):60–5.
20. Orlefors H, Sundin A, Ahlstrom H, et al. Positron emission tomography with 5-hydroxytryprophan in neuroendocrine tumors. J Clin Oncol 1998;16(7):2534–41.
21. Orlefors H, Sundin A, Garske U, et al. Whole-body (11)C-5-hydroxytryptophan positron emission tomography as a universal imaging technique for neuroendocrine tumors: comparison with somatostatin receptor scintigraphy and computed tomography. J Clin Endocrinol Metab 2005;90(6):3392–400.
22. Boellaard R, O'Doherty MJ, Weber WA, et al. FDG PET and PET/CT: EANM procedure guidelines for tumour PET imaging: version 1.0. Eur J Nucl Med Mol Imaging 2010;37(1):181–200.
23. Bombardieri E, Giammarile F, Aktolun C, et al. 131I/123I-metaiodobenzylguanidine (mIBG) scintigraphy: procedure guidelines for tumour imaging. Eur J Nucl Med Mol Imaging 2010;37(12):2436–46.

# Preclinical Studies of SPECT and PET Tracers for NET

Maarten Brom, PhD*, Otto Boerman, PhD,
Martin Gotthardt, MD, PhD, Wim J.G. Oyen, MD, PhD

## KEYWORDS

- Preclinical • Positron Emission Tomography • Single Photon Emission Computed Tomography
- Gastrin • Exendin • Bombesin • Animal models

## KEY POINTS

- Radiolabeled somatostatin analogues have been successfully used for the detection, staging, and treatment of neuroendocrine tumors (NETs). Based on the success achieved with somatostatin analogues and increasing knowledge of other peptide receptors expressed on NETs, other radiolabeled peptide analogues were developed for targeting of NETs.
- Several Exendin-, CCK/gastrin-, and bombesin-based analogues were labeled with a wide variety of radionuclides for SPECT or PET and were subsequently analyzed in vitro and in vivo in animal models for their stability, receptor affinity, in vivo tumor targeting, and pharmacokinetics. Some of these tracers have been translated in clinical studies, but usually still in small numbers of patients.
- Although some of these studies showed encouraging results and improved detection of certain tumor types that were not detected by conventional methods, clinical studies with larger numbers of patients must determine the added value of these techniques and the potential for use in routine clinical practice.

## INTRODUCTION

Neuroendocrine tumors (NETs) are tumors originating from endocrine cells and are characterized by the presence of secretory granules and the ability to produce biogenic amines and polypeptide hormones.[1] These tumors are derived from endocrine glands such as the adrenal medulla, pituitary, parathyroid, endocrine islets of the pancreas and thyroid as well as dispersed endocrine cells between the exocrine tissue of the respiratory and digestive system.[2] Most NETs are slow-growing tumors (well-differentiated NETs), whereas occasionally highly aggressive and very malignant tumors are observed (poorly differentiated NETs).[3] The outcome of the disease largely depends on early tumor detection. Molecular imaging is a promising method for the detection of tumors as well as NETs. Somatostatin receptor scintigraphy

is the most successful example of molecular imaging of NET that has progressed to large-scale clinical application. For staging and therapy monitoring of NETs, somatostatin targeting can be considered the detection method of choice. However, because of the heterogenous nature of NET, the detection rate in some tumor types is limited. Several other receptors and targets for molecular imaging and staging of these tumors have been proposed, such as the glucagon-like peptide-1 receptor (GLP-1R), cholecystokinin CCK/gastrin receptor, and gastrin releasing peptide receptor (GRPR).[4,5] The respective ligands exendin, CCK/gastrin, and bombesin were extensively studied in preclinical models and some of these tracers have already been tested in clinical studies. Despite these efforts, no new tracer, other than octreotide analogues, for the detection and staging of NETs, has reached the stage of standard clinical

Department of Nuclear Medicine, Radboud University Nijmegen Medical Centre, PO Box 9101, 6500 HB Nijmegen, The Netherlands
* Corresponding author.
E-mail address: m.brom@nucmed.umcn.nl

PET Clin 9 (2014) 63–69
http://dx.doi.org/10.1016/j.cpet.2013.08.012
1556-8598/14/$ – see front matter © 2014 Elsevier Inc. All rights reserved.

routine. In this review the efforts in preclinical studies to develop new positron emission tomography (PET) and single photon emission computed tomography (SPECT) tracers for the detection of NET are summarized. This review focuses on the most recent results on the development of exendin, CCK/gastrin, and bombesin-based radiopharmaceuticals and subsequent in vitro and in vivo characterization.

## EXENDIN

Insulinomas, mainly benign tumors derived from pancreatic β cells, are relatively rare. However, this tumor causes severe clinical symptoms because of the excessive production of insulin, resulting in sometimes life-threatening hypoglycemia. Detection of these tumors is challenging due to their small size and poor contrast to the surrounding pancreatic tissue on magnetic resonance imaging and computed tomography (CT). Somatostatin receptor scintigraphy, the gold standard for detection of NET, is not very well suited for detection of insulinomas because of the low incidence and density of somatostatin receptor subtype 2 and 5.[5,6] The GLP-1R is abundantly expressed in insulinomas and therefore potentially a better target for detecting insulinomas.[5] Because the natural ligand GLP-1 is rapidly degraded in plasma,[7] the stable agonists exendin-3 and exendin-4 are more suitable for GLP-1R targeting in vivo. First results with exendin-3, labeled [123]I, showed better in vitro and in vivo targeting compared with iodinated GLP-1.[7] However, the rapid washout of radioiodine from the cells after lysosomal degradation of the internalized compound results in low target-to-background ratios. Labeling with a radiometal of ligands conjugated with a chelator leads to high accumulation of the radiometal after internalization, because the radiometal-chelator complex is retained in the cell after internalization and catabolization. [111]In-labeled diethylenetriamene pentaacetate (DTPA)-exendin-4 showed efficient accumulation in GLP-1R-positive organs (pancreas, stomach, duodenum, and lung) in Wistar rats and BALB/c nude mice,[8] suggesting the feasibility to detect insulinomas by SPECT with this tracer. Wild and colleagues[9] showed excellent visualization of insulinomas in the pancreas of Rip1Tag2 mice by SPECT after injection of [111]In-DTPA-exendin-4. The tumor uptake of [111]In-DTPA-exendin-4 in this mouse model, that spontaneously develops insulinomas, was extremely high (287 ± 62% ID/g). Later, [68]Ga-labeled exendin was developed and characterized in the same model as well as in subcutaneous INS-1 cells (a rat insulinoma cell line) (**Fig. 1**).[10,11] Both studies showed similar in vivo targeting characteristics and the tumors were clearly visualized by PET. The extremely high accumulation of radiometal-chelate exendin-based tracers in the kidneys is caused by highly efficient reabsorption of the peptide (or its fragments) in the proximal tubules of the kidneys probably through the megalin/cubilin scavenger receptor system.[12] This high renal accumulation could hamper the visualization of lesions in close vicinity to the kidneys. Several attempts to reduce the kidney

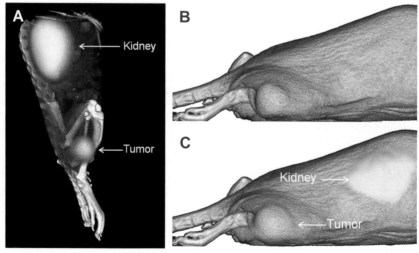

**Fig. 1.** (*A*) Lateral view of a maximum intensity projection of a PET image fused with CT of a BALB/c nude mouse with a subcutaneous INS-1 tumor after injection of [68]Ga-DOTA-exendin-3. (*B*) Surface rendering of the CT image and the overlay (*C*) with the [68]Ga-DOTA-exendin-3 PET image. Efficient accumulation is observed in the tumor on the hind leg of the mouse as well as accumulation in the kidney. Images were acquired 1 hour p.i.

accumulation, which is a general phenomenon for radiometal-labeled peptides, resulted in a marked reduction in kidney uptake. However, for [111]In-labeled exendin a maximum reduction of kidney accumulation of approximately only 50% was achieved by co-injection of a combination the gelatin-based plasma expender Gelofusin and polyglutamic acid.[13] Moreover, polyglutamic acid is not approved for clinical use and the use of Gelofusin alone resulted in a reduction of kidney uptake of only 20%.[13] Therefore, there is still a need to develop methods for effective reduction of the kidney uptake of radiolabeled exendin. Recently, exendin-4 and a stabilized GLP-1 analogue were labeled with [18]F through a maleimide-based prosthetic group (N-2-(4-[18]F-fluorobenzamido)ethyl-maleimide).[14,15] These [18]F-labeled analogues showed a markedly reduced kidney uptake resulting in better target-to-background ratios.

Several clinical studies and case reports suggest additional value of SPECT and PET with radiolabeled exendin for the detection of occult insulinomas.[16,17] However, a recent study showed that malignant insulinomas often lack GLP-1 receptors but often express somatostatin receptors, which could be targeted therapeutically.[18]

## GASTRIN

The CCK receptor family consists of 3 types: the CCK1 receptor (formerly known as CCK-A), CCK2 receptor (formerly known as CCK-B), and a splice variant of the CCK2 receptor CCK2i4sv.[19] CCK receptors have been identified in tumors and various normal tissues.[5,20] CCK2 receptors in particular are found on several tumor types with an extremely high expression on medullary thyroid carcinoma.[21] Furthermore, expression was found in astrocytomas and stromal ovarian cancer. CCK2i4sv is mainly expressed in colorectal and pancreatic cancer, but the expression level might be too low for detection of the tumor with radioactive tracers binding to this receptor.[22] Moreover, no specific tracer to target the splice variant only is available at the moment. The CCK1 receptor is hardly expressed in human tumors. Based on these observations of receptor expression, radiotracers for targeting the CCK2 receptor have been developed based on the regulatory peptides CCK and gastrin that specifically bind to the CCK2 receptor. The development and characterization of CCK-based and gastrin-based tracers have been extensively reviewed by Laverman and colleagues.[23]

Gotthardt and colleagues[24,25] showed added value of gastrin receptor scintigraphy especially in medullary thyroid carcinoma, as well as in

carcinoid and other NETs. The peptide used for these studies was a minigastrin analogue (MG0) conjugated with 1,4,7,10-tetraazacyclodo-decane-1,4,7,10-tetraacetic acid (DOTA) and labeled with [111]In, characterized by very high affinity for the CCK2 receptor and high in vivo accumulation in CCK2 receptor-positive tissues. The uptake of this tracer in CCK2 receptor-positive tumor is higher than that of tracer based on the CCK peptide. The major drawback of MG0 is the very high accumulation in the kidneys, due to efficient absorption in the proximal tubules of the kidneys, probably due to the presence of the N-terminal penta-glutamic acid sequence (**Fig. 2**). Removal of this penta-glutamic acid sequence results in lower accumulation in the kidneys, but unfortunately also in lower accumulation on CCK2 receptor-positive tumors, probably due to lower in vivo stability of these analogues. To reduce kidney uptake of MG0, Béhé and colleagues[26] showed that co-injection of polyglutamic acid efficiently blocks the kidney uptake of [111]In-MG0. Furthermore, comparison of 12 minigastrin-based radiotracers by a collaborative effort of several European research groups revealed a peptide (PP-F-11) that showed excellent in vivo characteristics: very efficient accumulation in the CCK2 receptor-positive tumor and low retention in the kidneys.[27-29] In this MG0-based peptide the N-terminal pentaglutamic acid sequence are replaced by 6 D-glutamic acid residues.[30] This

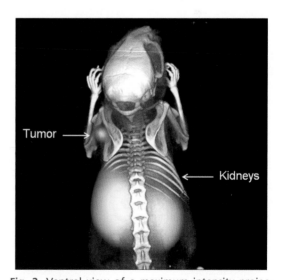

**Fig. 2.** Ventral view of a maximum intensity projection of a PET image of a BALB/c nude mouse with a subcutaneous AR42J tumor on the left shoulder after injection of [68]Ga-DOTA-MG0. The image was fused with CT for anatomic correlation. The tumor is clearly visible as well as the high accumulation in the kidneys. Images were acquired 1 hour p.i.

peptide holds great potential for preclinical as well as clinical detection of CCK2 receptor-positive tumor by PET and SPECT as well as therapy due to the low accumulation in the kidneys.

Recently, cyclic mingastrin analogues were produced aiming to obtain more stable gastrin-based tracers and in this way improve the in vivo targeting of CCK2 receptor-positive tumors. The authors showed high affinity and in vivo tumor uptake of the cyclic peptides labeled with [111]In or [68]Ga and were able to visualize subcutaneous CCK2 receptor-positive AR42J tumors. This study suggests that dimerization of gastrin analogues is a promising method to improve the in vitro and in vivo characteristics of gastrin analogues.

## BOMBESIN

Bombesin is a 14-amino-acid peptide of amphibian origin that together with its human counterpart GRP binds to GRPR. Besides physiologic effects as a brain-gut peptide, this class of peptides also plays an important role in cancer[31,32] as it was shown that tumor cell lines as well as human tumors can synthesize GRP.[33] The excreted peptides probably stimulate tumor growth by binding to bombesin receptors expressed on the tumor cell surface.[31–34] The bombesin receptor family consists of at least 4 subtypes: the neuromedin B (BB1), GRP receptor (BB2), BB3, and BB4 receptor.[35–38] The GRPR is most frequently overexpressed in several tumor types, such as prostate and breast carcinoma, small cell lung cancer, renal cell carcinoma, and gastrointestinal stromal tumors.[4,20,39] Because the GRPR is most frequently expressed in human tumors, this receptor and its respective ligands have been extensively characterized. Mostly the full-length bombesin or the truncated form was used for in vitro and in vivo targeting of the GRPR. Since the late 1990s many bombesin-based tracers were developed and labeled with a wide variety of radionuclides, such as [99m]Tc, [111]In, [67]Ga, for SPECT, [68]Ga, [64]Cu, and [18]F for PET, or [177]Lu for therapeutic purposes.[23] Major efforts have been underway to overcome the hepatobiliary clearance of bombesin, resulting in high uptake in the gastrointestinal tract, which obscures uptake in abdominal lesions. These efforts resulted in bombesin-based tracers with excellent receptor targeting properties combined with renal excretion of the tracer; some of these tracers were successfully used in clinical studies.[23]

More recently, a 1,4,7-triazacyclononane-N,N',N''-triacetic acid (NOTA)-conjugated bombesin antagonist was developed that was labeled with [111]In and [68]Ga.[40] NOTA was conjugated to the bombesin antagonist [D-Phe[6], Sta[13], Leu[14]] bombesin[6–14] via a diethylene glycol (PEG$_2$) ester to decrease hydrophilicity. Both the [111]In-labeled and the [68]Ga-labeled compound showed high labeling stability and high binding affinity and specificity for the GRPR. Studies in mice showed efficient accumulation in subcutaneous PC3 tumors combined with rapid clearance via the kidney, leading to excellent target-to-background ratios.[40] The subcutaneous PC3 tumor could be visualized by gamma camera (for the [111]In-labeled compound) or microPET (for the [68]Ga-labeled compound) as early as 1 hour after injection of the compounds. Another study with a bombesin antagonist showed influence of the chelator on the receptor affinity and in vivo tumor targeting.[41] This study described the conjugation of the chelators DOTA, 6-carboxy-1,4,7,11-tetraazaundecane (N4), 1,4,7-triazacyclononane, 1-glutaric acid-4,7 acetic acid, and 4,11-bis(carboxymethyl)-1,4,8,11-tetraazabicyclo[6.6.2]hexadecane to the bombesin antagonist AR (PEG4-D-Phe-Gln-Trp-Ala-Val-Gly-His-Sta-Leu-NH2) for labeling with [111]In, [99m]Tc, [68]Ga, and [64]Cu, respectively. All 4 conjugates showed high binding affinity in vitro in PC3 cells and retained their antagonistic properties. Also tumor targeting properties in nude mice with subcutaneous PC3 tumors were very good with high tumor uptake and rapid washout from nontarget tissues. The [64]Cu-labeled compound especially showed excellent imaging properties, favorable over the other conjugates, indicating the influence of the chelator on the receptor affinity. In line with these finding Fournier and colleagues[42] showed that the complex radiometal influences the receptor affinity and pharmacokinetics, as studied by [68]Ga and [64]Cu bombesin analogues. The same group designed bombesin dimers for improved targeting of the GRPR. The NOTA-conjugated bombesin dimers were labeled with [64]Cu and compared with the respective [64]Cu-labeled monomer. Both the monomer and the dimer were suitable for visualization of subcutaneous PC-3 tumors in nude mice with an improved retention of the dimer in the tumor.

Zhang and colleagues[43] studied the effect of the charge on the receptor affinity and showed that a positively charged bombesin agonist had a significantly higher affinity to the human GRPR. Replacement of the Nle[14] with a Met and the deletion of D-Tyr[6] further increased the affinity 6-fold. Subcutaneous PC-3 tumors in nude mice were clearly visualized by microPET after injection of this [64]Cu-labeled compound. However, the tumor uptake of this compound was much lower than that of the [64]Cu-labeled bombesin antagonist as reported in the previously mentioned study.[41] Dijkgraaf and colleagues[44] described the rapid and efficient labeling of a bombesin agonist with $^{18}$F with a 1-pot, 1-step synthesis based on the Al$^{18}$F labeling method.[45–47] The $^{18}$F-labeled agonist accumulated in subcutaneous PC-3 tumors in nude mice that could be detected by microPET. Although the labeled compound is hydrophilic and cleared via the kidneys, considerable intestinal uptake was observed in the PET images making detection of abdominal lesions with this compound difficult.

Preclinical studies with the DOTA-conjugated bombesin antagonist Sarabesin labeled with $^{68}$Ga showed very high accumulation in subcutaneous PC-3 tumors 4 hours post injection (p.i). The long retention in the tumors led to very good target-to-background ratios 24 p.i. and good visualization of the tumors by PET.[48] The results of the first clinical trials in patients with prostate and breast cancer with this tracer were promising.[48,49]

Patil and colleagues[50] used the strategy of bispecific antibodies to target GRPR expressing tumors and to increase the target-to-background ratio. This group linked either the intact anti-DTPA antibody or the Fab' fragment to bombesin for GRPR-specific targeting. They used the directly labeled antibody and Fab' fragment to determine the "pretargeting time" and subsequently determine the detection of subcutaneous PC3 tumors in SCID with the pretargeting method. Twenty-four hours after injection of the bispecific antibody or 8 hours after injection of the Fab' fragment, $^{111}$In- or $^{99m}$Tc-labeled DTPA-succinyl polylysine (DSPL) (respectively) was injected intravenously. Subcutaneous PC3 tumors of 2 to 3 mm could be visualized after injection of radiolabeled DSPL after pretargeting with the intact antibody or Fab' fragment 1 to 3 hours after injection with excellent tumor uptake at 240-hours p.i. Tumor imaging with the bispecific Fab' fragment with $^{99m}$Tc-DSPL was superior to the combination of the intact antibody with $^{111}$In-DSPL. The specificity for the GRPR was validated by blocking with bombesin or by pretargeting with the anti-DTPA antibody (not linked to bombesin).

## SUMMARY

Radiolabeled somatostatin analogues have been successfully used for the detection, staging, and treatment of NETs. Based on the success achieved with somatostatin analogues and increasing knowledge of other peptide receptors expressed on NETs, other radiolabeled peptide analogues were developed for targeting NETs. Several Exendin-, CCK/gastrin-, and bombesin-based analogues were labeled with a wide variety of radionuclides for SPECT or PET and were subsequently analyzed in vitro and in vivo in animals models for their stability, receptor affinity, in vivo tumor targeting, and pharmacokinetics. Some of these tracers have been translated in clinical studies, but usually still in small numbers of patients. Although some of these studies showed encouraging results and improved detection of certain tumor types that were not detected by conventional methods, clinical studies with larger numbers of patients must determine the added value of these techniques and the potential for use in routine clinical practice.

## REFERENCES

1. Rufini V, Calcagni ML, Baum RP. Imaging of neuroendocrine tumors. Semin Nucl Med 2006;36(3): 228–47.
2. Kaltsas GA, Besser GM, Grossman AB. The diagnosis and medical management of advanced neuroendocrine tumors. Endocr Rev 2004;25(3): 458–511.
3. Solcia E, Kloeppel G, Sobin L. World Health Organization international histological classification of tumours: histological typing of endocrine tumours: second edition. Clin Endocrinol 2000; 53(2):259.
4. Reubi JC. Peptide receptors as molecular targets for cancer diagnosis and therapy. Endocr Rev 2003;24(4):389–427.
5. Reubi JC, Waser B. Concomitant expression of several peptide receptors in neuroendocrine tumours: molecular basis for in vivo multireceptor tumour targeting. Eur J Nucl Med Mol Imaging 2003;30(5):781–93.
6. Modlin IM, Tang LH. Approaches to the diagnosis of gut neuroendocrine tumors: the last word (today). Gastroenterology 1997;112(2):583–90.
7. Gotthardt M, Fischer M, Naeher I, et al. Use of the incretin hormone glucagon-like peptide-1 (GLP-1) for the detection of insulinomas: initial experimental results. Eur J Nucl Med Mol Imaging 2002;29(5): 597–606.
8. Gotthardt M, Lalyko G, van Eerd-Vismale J, et al. A new technique for in vivo imaging of specific GLP-1 binding sites: first results in small rodents. Regul Pept 2006;137(3):162–7.
9. Wild D, Behe M, Wicki A, et al. [Lys40(Ahx-DTPA-111In)NH2]exendin-4, a very promising ligand for glucagon-like peptide-1 (GLP-1) receptor targeting. J Nucl Med 2006;47(12):2025–33.
10. Wild D, Wicki A, Mansi R, et al. Exendin-4-based radiopharmaceuticals for glucagonlike peptide-1 receptor PET/CT and SPECT/CT. J Nucl Med 2010;51(7):1059–67.
11. Brom M, Oyen WJ, Joosten L, et al. 68Ga-labelled exendin-3, a new agent for the detection of

insulinomas with PET. Eur J Nucl Med Mol Imaging 2010;37(7):1345–55.

12. Vegt E, Melis M, Eek A, et al. Renal uptake of different radiolabelled peptides is mediated by megalin: SPECT and biodistribution studies in megalin-deficient mice. Eur J Nucl Med Mol Imaging 2011;38(4):623–32.

13. Gotthardt M, van Eerd-Vismale J, Oyen WJ, et al. Indication for different mechanisms of kidney uptake of radiolabeled peptides. J Nucl Med 2007; 48(4):596–601.

14. Gao H, Niu G, Yang M, et al. PET of insulinoma using (1)(8)F-FBEM-EM3106B, a new GLP-1 analogue. Mol Pharm 2011;8(5):1775–82.

15. Kiesewetter DO, Gao H, Ma Y, et al. 18F-radiolabeled analogs of exendin-4 for PET imaging of GLP-1 in insulinoma. Eur J Nucl Med Mol Imaging 2012;39(3):463–73.

16. Christ E, Wild D, Forrer F, et al. Glucagon-like peptide-1 receptor imaging for localization of insulinomas. J Clin Endocrinol Metab 2009;94(11): 4398–405.

17. Wild D, Macke H, Christ E, et al. Glucagon-like peptide 1-receptor scans to localize occult insulinomas. N Engl J Med 2008;359(7):766–8.

18. Wild D, Christ E, Caplin ME, et al. Glucagon-like peptide-1 versus somatostatin receptor targeting reveals 2 distinct forms of malignant insulinomas. J Nucl Med 2011;52(7):1073–8.

19. Hellmich MR, Rui XL, Hellmich HL, et al. Human colorectal cancers express a constitutively active cholecystokinin-B/gastrin receptor that stimulates cell growth. J Biol Chem 2000; 275(41):32122–8.

20. Reubi JC, Korner M, Waser B, et al. High expression of peptide receptors as a novel target in gastrointestinal stromal tumours. Eur J Nucl Med Mol Imaging 2004;31(6):803–10.

21. Reubi JC, Waser B. Unexpected high incidence of cholecystokinin-B/gastrin receptors in human medullary thyroid carcinomas. Int J Cancer 1996;67(5): 644–7.

22. Korner M, Waser B, Reubi JC, et al. CCK(2) receptor splice variant with intron 4 retention in human gastrointestinal and lung tumours. J Cell Mol Med 2010;14(4):933–43.

23. Laverman P, Sosabowski JK, Boerman OC, et al. Radiolabelled peptides for oncological diagnosis. Eur J Nucl Med Mol Imaging 2012;39(Suppl 1): S78–92.

24. Gotthardt M, Behe MP, Beuter D, et al. Improved tumour detection by gastrin receptor scintigraphy in patients with metastasised medullary thyroid carcinoma. Eur J Nucl Med Mol Imaging 2006;33(11): 1273–9.

25. Gotthardt M, Behe MP, Grass J, et al. Added value of gastrin receptor scintigraphy in

comparison to somatostatin receptor scintigraphy in patients with carcinoids and other neuroendocrine tumours. Endocr Relat Cancer 2006;13(4): 1203–11.

26. Béhé M, Kluge G, Becker W, et al. Use of polyglutamic acids to reduce uptake of radiometal-labeled minigastrin in the kidneys. J Nucl Med 2005;46(6): 1012–5.

27. Aloj L, Aurilio M, Rinaldi V, et al. Comparison of the binding and internalization properties of 12 DOTA-coupled and (1)(1)(1)In-labelled CCK2/gastrin receptor binding peptides: a collaborative project under COST Action BM0607. Eur J Nucl Med Mol Imaging 2011;38(8):1417–25.

28. Laverman P, Joosten L, Eek A, et al. Comparative biodistribution of 12(1)(1)(1)In-labelled gastrin/CCK2 receptor-targeting peptides. Eur J Nucl Med Mol Imaging 2011;38(8):1410–6.

29. Ocak M, Helbok A, Rangger C, et al. Comparison of biological stability and metabolism of CCK2 receptor targeting peptides, a collaborative project under COST BM0607. Eur J Nucl Med Mol Imaging 2011;38(8):1426–35.

30. Kolenc-Peitl P, Mansi R, Tamma M, et al. Highly improved metabolic stability and pharmacokinetics of indium-111-DOTA-gastrin conjugates for targeting of the gastrin receptor. J Med Chem 2011; 54(8):2602–9.

31. Kroog GS, Jensen RT, Battey JF. Mammalian bombesin receptors. Med Res Rev 1995;15(5): 389–417.

32. Cuttitta F, Carney DN, Mulshine J, et al. Bombesin-like peptides can function as autocrine growth factors in human small-cell lung cancer. Nature 1985; 316(6031):823–6.

33. Moody TW, Pert CB, Gazdar AF, et al. High levels of intracellular bombesin characterize human small-cell lung carcinoma. Science 1981;214(4526): 1246–8.

34. Moody TW, Carney DN, Cuttitta F, et al. High affinity receptors for bombesin/GRP-like peptides on human small cell lung cancer. Life Sci 1985;37(2): 105–13.

35. Nagalla SR, Barry BJ, Creswick KC, et al. Cloning of a receptor for amphibian [Phe13]bombesin distinct from the receptor for gastrin-releasing peptide: identification of a fourth bombesin receptor subtype (BB4). Proc Natl Acad Sci U S A 1995; 92(13):6205–9.

36. Fathi Z, Corjay MH, Shapira H, et al. BRS-3: a novel bombesin receptor subtype selectively expressed in testis and lung carcinoma cells. J Biol Chem 1993;268(8):5979–84.

37. Wada E, Way J, Shapira H, et al. cDNA cloning, characterization, and brain region-specific expression of a neuromedin-B-preferring bombesin receptor. Neuron 1991;6(3):421–30.

38. Spindel ER, Giladi E, Brehm P, et al. Cloning and functional characterization of a complementary DNA encoding the murine fibroblast bombesin/gastrin-releasing peptide receptor. Mol Endocrinol 1990;4(12):1956–63.

39. Reubi JC, Wenger S, Schmuckli-Maurer J, et al. Bombesin receptor subtypes in human cancers: detection with the universal radioligand (125)I-[D-TYR(6), beta-ALA(11), PHE(13), NLE(14)] bombesin(6-14). Clin Cancer Res 2002;8(4):1139–46.

40. Varasteh Z, Velikyan I, Lindeberg G, et al. Synthesis and characterization of a high-affinity NOTA-conjugated bombesin antagonist for GRPR-targeted tumor imaging. Bioconjug Chem 2013. [Epub ahead of print].

41. Abiraj K, Mansi R, Tamma ML, et al. Bombesin antagonist-based radioligands for translational nuclear imaging of gastrin-releasing peptide receptor-positive tumors. J Nucl Med 2011;52(12):1970–8.

42. Fournier P, Dumulon-Perreault V, Ait-Mohand S, et al. Novel radiolabeled peptides for breast and prostate tumor PET imaging: (64)Cu/and (68)Ga/NOTA-PEG-[D-Tyr(6), betaAla(11), Thi(13), Nle(14)] BBN(6-14). Bioconjug Chem 2012;23(8):1687–93.

43. Zhang H, Abiraj K, Thorek DL, et al. Evolution of bombesin conjugates for targeted PET imaging of tumors. PLoS One 2012;7(9):e44046.

44. Dijkgraaf I, Franssen GM, McBride WJ, et al. PET of tumors expressing gastrin-releasing peptide receptor with an 18F-labeled bombesin analog. J Nucl Med 2012;53(6):947–52.

45. D'Souza CA, McBride WJ, Sharkey RM, et al. High-yielding aqueous 18F-labeling of peptides via Al18F chelation. Bioconjug Chem 2011;22(9):1793–803.

46. Laverman P, McBride WJ, Sharkey RM, et al. A novel facile method of labeling octreotide with (18)F-fluorine. J Nucl Med 2010;51(3):454–61.

47. Schoffelen R, Sharkey RM, Goldenberg DM, et al. Pretargeted immuno-positron emission tomography imaging of carcinoembryonic antigen-expressing tumors with a bispecific antibody and a 68Ga- and 18F-labeled hapten peptide in mice with human tumor xenografts. Mol Cancer Ther 2010;9(4):1019–27.

48. Maina T, de Jong M, Charalambidis D, et al. [67/68Ga]Sarabesin 3: preclinical evaluation in GRPR-expressing models - first successful clinical PET/CT imaging of prostate cancer metastases. J Nucl Med Meeting Abstracts 2013;54(2_MeetingAbstracts):447.

49. Bergsma H, Kulkarni H, Mueller D, et al. PET/CT imaging with a novel 68Ga-labelled GRP-receptor antagonist, Sarabesin 3. First clinical data in patients with prostate and breast cancer. J Nucl Med Meeting Abstracts 2013;54(2_MeetingAbstracts):280.

50. Patil V, Gada K, Panwar R, et al. Imaging small human prostate cancer xenografts after pretargeting with bispecific bombesin-antibody complexes and targeting with high specific radioactivity labeled polymer-drug conjugates. Eur J Nucl Med Mol Imaging 2012;39(5):824–39.

# Yttrium-Based Therapy for Neuroendocrine Tumors

Lisa Bodei, MD, PhD[a], Marta Cremonesi, PhD[b],
Giovanni Paganelli, MD[a],*

## KEYWORDS

- $^{90}$Y-DOTATOC • Peptide receptor radionuclide therapy • PRRT • Neuroendocrine tumors
- Dosimetry

## KEY POINTS

- Peptide receptor radionuclide therapy (PRRT) finds its main indication in the treatment of inoperable or metastasized neuroendocrine tumors, and G1 and G2 tumors are the ideal candidates.
- After 17 years of experience, PRRT with $^{90}$Y-peptides are generally well tolerated; in addition, acute side effects are usually mild.
- Objective responses to $^{90}$Y-peptides are registered in 10% to 34% of patients, with a significant impact on survival and quality of life.

## INTRODUCTION

Peptide receptor radionuclide therapy (PRRT) finds its main indication in the treatment of inoperable or metastasized neuroendocrine tumors (NETs), particularly of the gastroenteropancreatic (GEP) tract. Well/moderately differentiated G1 and G2 tumors are the ideal candidates.[1]

PRRT was introduced in clinical practice in 1994 as the next logical step of the in vivo localization of a metastatic neuroendocrine tumor with the radiolabeled somatostatin analogue [$^{111}$In-DTPA0-D-Phe1]-octreotide.[2]

Subsequently, many patients have been treated with high-dose [$^{111}$In-DTPA0-D-Phe1]-octreotide, exploiting the Auger and conversion electrons of $^{111}$In. Partial remissions, however, have been observed only exceptionally.[3]

Higher-energy and longer-range emitters, such as the pure beta emitter $^{90}$Y, seemed more suitable for therapeutic purposes. The higher energy (maximum 2.2 MeV) and penetration range ($R_{95}$ 5.7 mm) of β particles from $^{90}$Y are advantageous, with a direct killing of somatostatin receptor-positive cells and a cross fire effect that hits nearby receptor-negative tumor cells. A new analogue name, Tyr$^3$-octreotide, with a similar pattern of affinity for somatostatin receptors was developed at the University of Basel for its high hydrophilicity, simple labeling with $^{111}$In and $^{90}$Y, and tight binding to the bifunctional chelator DOTA (1,4,7,10-tetra-azacyclododecane-N,N',N'',N'''-tetra-acetic acid).[4,5]

[$^{90}$Y-DOTA$^0$,Tyr$^3$]-octreotide or $^{90}$Y-DOTATOC was first administered in patients affected by metastatic neuroendocrine tumors in 1996. The excellent symptomatic and objective response following several cycles of $^{90}$Y-DOTATOC therapy led to high expectations regarding the potential of PRRT for other patients with NET tumors.[6]

Other clinical experiences have been carried out with $^{90}$Y-lanreotide, a different somatostatin receptor agonist.[7]

Funding Sources: The authors have nothing to disclose.
Conflict of Interest: The authors have nothing to disclose.
[a] Division of Nuclear Medicine, European Institute of Oncology, via Ripamonti 435, 20141 Milan, Italy;
[b] Division of Medical Physics, European Institute of Oncology, via Ripamonti 435, 20141 Milan, Italy
* Corresponding author.
E-mail address: divisione.medicinanucleare@ieo.it

pet.theclinics.com

Somatostatin analogues represent, to date, the prototype and the most successful paradigm of radiopeptide therapy because of the fortunate discovery of a successful class of synthetic peptides, such as octreotide and its variants, and to the inhibiting properties of somatostatin and its analogues, which induce few and limited side effects. The success of the clinical application of the octapeptide somatostatin analogues, such as octreotide, and, subsequently, of their radiolabeled counterparts, such as the [$^{90}$Y-DOTA$^0$,Tyr$^3$]-modified form, was caused by their high affinity for somatostatin receptors subtype 2 (sst2) and moderate affinity for subtype 5 (sst5), perfectly tailored to the prevalent expression of sst2 and sst5 in neuroendocrine tumors.

Since 2000, the new analogue DOTATATE ([DOTA$^0$,Tyr$^3$,Thr$^8$]-octreotide or octreotate), with a 9-fold higher affinity for sst2 as compared with [DOTA$^0$,Tyr$^3$]-octreotide, was introduced in clinical use for its easy labeling to the beta- and gamma-emitting radionuclide lutetium-177.[8]

Owing to its efficacy and reasonably acceptable toxicity, since its introduction, PRRT with $^{90}$Y-DOTATOC or $^{177}$Lu-DOTATATE has been used in several clinical trials over the following years in many centers, mainly in Europe but also in the United States and Australia.

Seventeen years after its first introduction, despite the lack of homogeneity among the studies, PRRT can be regarded as efficient and reasonably safe.

## RADIOBIOLOGIC BASIS OF PRRT

From a dosimetric point of view, the efficacy of PRRT relies on a sufficient radioactivity concentration in tumors. This concentration is related to tumor receptor density as well as receptor affinity and pharmacokinetic characteristics of the radiopeptide used.[9] Predictive factors for tumor shrinkage are, in fact, a high uptake at basal somatostatin receptor imaging, with either Octreoscan or positron emission tomography (PET) with Ga-DOTA-peptides, and a small volume of liver metastases.[10,11] The uptake at basal somatostatin receptor imaging represents a rough estimate of the absorbed dose. The dose is, in fact, predictive of the tumor response.[12] Nevertheless, there is no well-defined threshold dose for tumor control but a certain probability over a range of doses.[13] Besides tumor dose, other modulating factors have to be considered, first of all radiosensitivity (which accounts for the individual, genetically based responsiveness to the treatment), repair, redistribution, reoxygenation, and repopulation (the so-called 5 Rs of radiobiology). Additionally, the nonuniformity of uptake (caused by variable receptor density, vascularization, and interstitial pressure) as well as the tumor volume and the number of clonogenic stem cells must be considered. Finally, the type of radionuclide used, its range, cross fire, and energy deposition within tumor lesions must be taken into account.

To understand the biologic basis of tissue damage after irradiation, we have to consider the type of tissue organization. Tissues may show rapid turnover, like bone marrow, mucosae, and most tumors, with a hierarchical organization, whereby stem cells produce precursors that, in turn, produce mature cells. Damage to these cells is typically acute (<90 days) and evident after the lifespan of the mature cell has elapsed. Acute damage may be reversible. Other tissues, like the kidney whose cells mostly die of senescence, show a slow turnover. In this case, damage is typically delayed and irreversible, associated with vascular changes, fibrosis, and atrophy. However, late effects may also occur in rapidly renewing tissues, such as myelo displastic syndrome (MDS) or acute leukemia, which may occur in irradiated patients.[14]

Kidney radiation toxicity is typically evident several months after irradiation because of the slow repair characteristics of renal cell.

PRRT is a form of continuous radiation delivery with a decreasing dose rate over time. The irradiation produces both lethal and sublethal damage that can be repaired during the irradiation itself, but the differential between creating new damage and the repairing depends on the specific dose rate at any particular time and on the repair capability of the tissue. Low-dose rates, as in PRRT, will spare normal tissues more than the tumor; this may allow benefits as in fractionation in external radiotherapy.[15]

The linear quadratic model interprets mathematically this differential sparing, and the biologic effective dose (BED) concept is used to quantify the biologic effects induced by different patterns of radiation delivery. This model has been recently revised for radionuclide therapy and has been applied in particular to PRRT with the intent of increasing the dose-response correlation.[16] Focusing on the kidney concern, the BED has proven to be a reliable predictor of renal toxicity, which is helpful in the implementation of individual treatment planning.[17] In PRRT, the BED has been shown to correlate with renal injury. However, BED is a relatively young concept applied to nuclear medicine and still has to be fully validated with a wider series of data.

The main radiobiological parameter required in such assessment is the tissue $\alpha/\beta$ ratio, which gives an indication of the sensitivity of a tumor or normal tissue cell to the effect of the dose rate (and/or fractionation) and is generally higher for tumors (5–25 Gy) than for late-responding normal tissues (2–5 Gy), such as the kidneys.

Interindividual variations in the risk of normal tissue complications are, therefore, substantial.[18]

For many tissues, including tumors, radiation damage will not be evident for days (eg, for the bone marrow) or months (eg, for the kidneys) until the cells attempt to divide. This phenomenon is related to the peculiar proliferation characteristics of the tissues. In tumors, the time necessary for shrinkage to be evident varies among different histotypes and even among tumors of the same histotype, according to the characteristics of the single lesion. The interval between therapy and volume reduction depends on the proportion of the stromal and cellular components, on the rate of removal of the cellular and noncellular material, on the cellular kinetics, and the tumor proliferation rate.[19]

From a radiobiological point of view, PRRT is able to induce various degrees of cell kill, depending on the dose delivered, the type of radiation used (eg, $^{90}Y$ or $^{177}Lu$), and the tumor volume. Tumor intrinsic characteristics like radiosensitivity, growth, and heterogeneity are other important parameters to consider for the response.[20] Tumor doses experimentally found as adequate to induce a significant shrinkage vary over a range of 120 to 150 Gy with $^{90}Y$-DOTATOC.[13]

## DISTINCTIVE FEATURES OF TUMOR IRRADIATION

The major task for PRRT is to deliver the maximal detrimental dose to the tumor while limiting the irradiation of normal organs as much as possible. Currently, the potential risk of kidney and red marrow limits the amount of radioactivity that may be administered. However, when tumor masses are irradiated with adequate doses, volume reduction may be observed.[13] Tumor remission is positively correlated with a high uptake at [$^{111}In$-DTPA$^0$]-octreotide scintigraphy.[12]

Nevertheless, the tumor dose does not only depend directly on the administered activity and the uptake versus time, namely, on the amount of energy released within the tumor, but also on its mass. Roughly, smaller masses have a higher chance of reduction because a higher absorbed dose is concentrated within their volume.

Another factor influencing tumor irradiation and, therefore, the response is the choice of the radionuclide. In particular, $^{90}Y$ particles are highly energetic and penetrating and lead to a better cross fire through the tumor, which is particularly valuable in larger tumors and when heterogeneous

receptor and/or activity distribution exists. The shorter half-life of $^{90}Y$ allows a higher dose rate. $^{177}Lu$, on the other hand, has lower energy and smaller particle range, allowing a better absorption in smaller tumors.[21]

Mathematical models showed that $^{177}Lu$ is more suitable for small tumors, with an optimal diameter of 2 mm, whereas $^{90}Y$ is more suitable in larger ones, with an optimal diameter of 34 mm. Theoretically, $^{90}Y$ seems, therefore, less appropriate for PRRT of small tumors because very small masses are not likely to absorb all the β-energy released in the tumor cells. As opposed to this, $^{177}Lu$ seems less ideal for larger tumors because of the lack of uniformity of activity distribution within the tumor mass. Finally, differences in the dose rate must be taken into account: the longer physical half-life of $^{177}Lu$ means a longer period needed to deliver the same dose as $^{90}Y$. This factor may allow more time for tumor repopulation.[22] A combination therapy with $^{90}Y$ and $^{177}Lu$, either simultaneously or in distinct settings, has been, therefore, suggested to overcome the difficulties of a real clinical situation of different-sized lesions. Nevertheless, clinical experiences are still limited.

Studies comparing the doses recorded at any cycle of PRRT showed that tumor uptake gradually reduced in subsequent cycles, most likely because of saturation or downregulation of the receptors. The contribution to the tumor absorbed dose diminished progressively (~35% of the cumulative dose being released at the first cycle, whereas ~15% at the fourth cycle), with the first 2 cycles having a major impact.[23] These findings are in agreement with the clinical outcomes shown by van Essen and colleagues[24] who observed lower antitumor effects from additional treatment after regular cycles in patients with a short time to progression.

## CLINICAL DOSIMETRY

If feasible, dosimetry of normal organs and tumor is a useful aid for patient selection and therapy planning.[1] In fact, there is wide variability among patients of the radiopeptide uptake of normal organs and tumor tissues related to varying somatostatin receptor densities on tumor cells and to factors such as tumor volume, interstitial pressure, and viability.

Tailoring PRRT according to dosimetry has been shown to be of great value in clinical practice and should replace the criteria of administering a fixed amount of radioactivity amount or an activity correct for the patients' body weight or surface. However, the method of collecting and analyzing data is crucial. In fact, if data are not available up to

2 effective half-lives ($\sim$4 days for $^{177}$Lu, $\sim$3 days for $^{90}$Y), the estimation of the kidney-absorbed dose is consistently influenced by the interpolation method. Moreover, using DOTATATE instead of DOTATOC causes a dose increase of 1.25 to 1.30.[25] Several investigators have explored the impact of using different 2-dimensional and 3-dimensional (3D) dosimetric methods.[23,26,27] These studies, focused on the kidneys, evidenced a typical 15% overestimate of planar as compared with 3D dosimetry, and about 10% differences with 3D dosimetry in relation to the volume of interest.

In PRRT with $^{90}$Y-peptides, dosimetry cannot be straightforwardly reconstructed from bremsstrahlung images, due to the lack of a gamma emission allowing a direct quantitative analysis. Therefore, 2 surrogate approaches have been developed, specifically the simulation with an $^{111}$In-labelled peptide, biochemically similar to the original one, and the simulation with the $^{86}$Y-labelled peptide, biochemically identical to the therapeutic counterpart.[28,29]

Although [$^{90}$Y-DOTA$^0$,Tyr$^3$]-octreotide (or -lanreotide or -octreotate) and its imageable counterpart [$^{111}$In-DOTA$^0$,Tyr$^3$]-octreotide (or -lanreotide or -octreotate) are not the same molecule, the latter has been used for dosimetric simulation based on the hypothesis that the similar physical and biologic half-lives yield comparable in vivo pharmacokinetics and biodistribution, especially concerning the renal uptake, which is thought to depend mainly on nonspecific phenomena. A drawback of this method is that the small structural modification caused by the metal replacement can possibly affect the somatostatin receptor binding affinity and, therefore, lead to a slight inaccuracy of the estimation of the renal uptake.[30]

The first results obtained with this method[28] showed a fast blood clearance (<1% injected activity in blood 10 hours p.i. post injection) and rapid urine elimination (52% $\pm$ 12% injected activity 4 hours p.i. and >70% 24 hours p.i.), therefore, indicating a low total body irradiation deriving from [$^{90}$Y-DOTA$^0$,Tyr$^3$]-octreotide. The in vivo stability of the radiopeptide, assessed both in urine and in plasma, seemed to be high; no degradation product was found in blood. According to biodistribution, the organs receiving the highest predicted absorbed doses, in a first series of 18 patients, include the spleen (7.6 $\pm$ 6.3 mGy/MBq), the kidneys (3.3 $\pm$ 2.2 mGy/MBq) and the tumor (1.4–31.0 mGy/MBq, mean 10). Enlarging the series to 30 patients, studied en blanc, before therapy, namely, without renal protection, a slightly higher value of kidney dose (3.9 $\pm$ 1.9 mGy/MBq) was observed.[31]

A thorough dosimetric study using the same chemical radiocompound, namely [DOTA$^0$,Tyr$^3$]-octreotide labeled with the positron emitter $^{86}$Y, was carried out in 24 patients.[32] PET with [$^{86}$Y-DOTA$^0$,Tyr$^3$]-octreotide offers substantial advantages in the spatial resolution and quantification. Nevertheless, the short half-life of the radionuclide leaves the interpretation of the later phases of the biokinetics to extrapolation. Despite the lack of an actual comparison study between the 2 simulation techniques, pharmacokinetic parameters were similar ($\sim$5% Injected Activity [I.A.] in plasma 5 hours p.i. and <1% after 24 hours), as well as the kidney dose (4.4 $\pm$ 1.0 mGy/MBq, in 4 patients), to the ones calculated with [$^{111}$In-DOTA$^0$,-Tyr$^3$]-octreotide (3.9 $\pm$ 1.9 Gy/GBq). The mean estimated tumor dose for $^{90}$Y was highly variable (1.5–177.1 Gy delivered by the maximum activities administered).

Recently, a new method of analyzing $^{90}$Y images for dosimetric purposes has been developed, therefore, allowing the omission of simulations with $^{111}$In or $^{86}$Y-imaging.[33,34]

## SAFETY PROFILE

After 17 years of experience, we can state that, from the safety point of view, PRRT with $^{90}$Y-peptides is generally well tolerated. Acute side effects are usually mild; some of them are related to the coadministration of amino acids, such as nausea (or more rarely vomit), and others are related to the radiopeptide, such as fatigue (commonly), or the exacerbation of an endocrine syndrome, which rarely occurs in functioning tumors. Chronic and permanent effects on target organs, particularly the kidneys and the bone marrow, are generally mild if the necessary precautions, such as fractionation and attention to specific risk factors, are taken (**Table 1**).[9,11,35–37]

Dosimetric studies indicated that it is possible to deliver elevated absorbed doses to the tumor while limiting the dose to organs, such as kidneys and bone marrow, to tolerance limits.

Although hematological toxicity mainly occurs immediately after PRRT and is usually mild and transient, permanent and severe bone marrow toxicity is usually a rare event after PRRT because the resulting bone marrow absorbed doses is, in general, less than the threshold of toxicity.[38] The delayed renal toxicity that may occur if the dose threshold is exceeded is permanent.

Results from the 2 Milan phase I studies, considering escalating activities from 1.11 GBq to 2.59 GBq per cycle without amino acid protection and from 2.96 to 5.55 GBq per cycle with amino acid coinfusion, indicated the maximum

**Table 1**
**Long-term toxicity after $^{90}$Y-DOTATOC in patients affected by NETs**

| Center | Patient Number | Follow-up (mo) | Renal Toxicity (Creatinine) | MDS | Leukemia |
|---|---|---|---|---|---|
| Milan | 40 | 19 | 10% Grade 1 | 0 | 0 |
| Basel | 41 | 15 | 0 | 0 | 0 |
| Basel | 39 | 6 | 3% Grade 2 | 0 | 0 |
| Multicenter | 58 | 18 | 3% Grade 4 | 1 | 0 |
| Copenhagen | 53 | 17 | 0 | 1 | 0 |
| Basel | 1109 | 23 | 9.2% Grade 3/4[a] | 1 | 1 |

[a] Toxicity grade measured on glomerular filtration rate.
*Data from* Refs.[11,35–37,50,56]

tolerated activity per cycle as 5.18 GBq, based mainly on acute hematological toxicity. The maximum cumulative activity, resulting from dosimetric estimates, was based mainly on the dosimetric burden to the kidneys and ranged between 10 and 15 GBq.[39]

## Kidney

In view of their marked radiosensitivity, the kidneys represent the critical organs after $^{90}$Y-DOTA-peptides at the radiation doses that are normally reached with PRRT. Renal irradiation arises from the proximal tubular reabsorption, following the glomerular filtration of the radiopeptide, and the resulting accumulation in the interstitium. Studies with external radiotherapy indicated a threshold of tolerance in the range of 23 to 27 Gy.[40]

However, the intrinsically different dose rate deriving from PRRT is expected to result in a different threshold of the absorbed dose. The recently introduced BED concept, which represents a sort of universal code to express the dose, regardless of the modality with which it was delivered, is more accurate in predicting toxicity. The renal BED threshold for toxicity after PRRT was indicated to be as high as 40 Gy.[16,17]

When using DOTATATE labeled with $^{90}$Y, it has to be pointed out that this peptide shows a longer residence time in the kidneys and this leads to even higher renal absorbed doses per unit of activity.[9,25,41]

Renal protection with positively charged amino acids, such as lysine or arginine, competitively inhibiting the radiopeptide reabsorption, is currently mandatory because it has been demonstrated that this strategy leads to a 9% to 53% reduction of the renal doses.[42,43] Prolonging the infusion time, thus covering more extensively the elimination phase through the kidneys, results in a further reduction of renal doses (up to 39% by prolonging infusion

over 10 hours and up to 65% by prolonging it over 2 days after radiopeptide administration).[31]

However, despite renal protection, a loss of renal function of variable degree, but generally mild, constantly occurs, with a median decline in creatinine clearance of 7.3% per year for $^{90}$Y-octreotide as opposed to a median 3.8% per year for $^{177}$Lu-octreotate.[44] This loss of renal function potentially leaves sensitive patients, or those with a limited renal function at therapy start, with an evident damage months after the end of PRRT.

However, cases of severe, end-stage renal damage are now rare. They mainly occurred at the beginning of the PRRT experience when very high activities were administered, especially in patients who have received more than 7.4 GBq/m$^2$, and when renal protection was not in use.[45]

Nephrotoxicity, in fact, is accelerated by other risk factors besides the dose resulting from the cumulative activity. Studies demonstrated that a higher and more persistent decline in creatinine clearance and the subsequent development of renal toxicity is likely to occur in those patients with risk factors for delayed renal toxicity, particularly long-standing and poorly controlled diabetes and hypertension. In a long-term evaluation of renal toxicity after PRRT in a group of 28 patients undergoing PRRT with dosimetric analysis, 23 of which were treated with $^{90}$Y-DOTATOC, toxicity on creatinine, according to the National Cancer Institute's criteria, occurred in 9 patients (7 grade 1, 1 grade 2, 1 grade 3). Creatinine clearance loss at 1 year was greater than 5% in 12 cases and greater than 10% in 8. A low 28-Gy BED threshold was observed in patients with risk factors (mainly hypertension and diabetes), whereas it was 40 Gy in patients without risk factors.[46]

In a retrospective series of 1109 patients treated with $^{90}$Y-DOTATOC at the University of Basel, 103 patients (9.2%) experienced grade 4 to 5 permanent renal toxicity.[11] Multivariable regression revealed that the initial kidney uptake was predictive for severe renal toxicity. However, this relatively high incidence could be related to the high administered activities per cycle (3.7 GBq/m$^2$ body surface, namely, activities of about 6.4 GBq per cycle in a standard man) and to the fact that patients with preexisting impairment of renal function were not excluded from PRRT. Moreover, the possible lack of use of amino acids in the first years of study also has to be considered.[45] These data indicate that hyperfractionating the therapy into multiple fractions with lower activity per cycle could be beneficial in terms of safety, which largely depends on the activity per cycle.

Clinical experience and dosimetric studies clearly indicate that the renal absorbed dose estimated by conventional dosimetry may not accurately correlate with the renal toxicity observed in patients treated with [$^{90}$Y-DOTA$^0$,Tyr$^3$]-octreotide. Additional parameters, such as patient-specific kidney volume and distribution of the radionuclide, seemed to give a better correlation with clinical effects.[17] The assessment of individual kidney volume by computed tomography (CT) scan yields a wide variability when compared with the standardized phantom. New CT-based techniques accounting for the difference in the placement of radioactivity within the kidneys seem more realistic.[47]

Unfortunately, at present, data from ex vivo autoradiography in humans regarding the activity distribution of radiolabeled somatostatin analogues are contradicting and not conclusive because the radioactivity distribution of $^{111}$In-pentetreotide was reported as inhomogeneously distributed, about 70% in the cortex and 30% in the medulla, whereas $^{90}$Y/$^{111}$In-DOTATOC was found to be homogeneously distributed in the cortical and medullary structures, without a significant gradient.[48,49] A possible explanation for these differences relies on the effect of amino acid protectors, used for therapy, which interfere with the natural distribution of peptides within the kidneys.

## Bone Marrow

From a hematological point of view, PRRT is generally well tolerated. Severe, World Health Organization (WHO) grade 3 or 4, toxicity does not occur in more than 13% of cases after $^{90}$Y-octreotide. Nevertheless, sporadic cases of MDS or even overt acute leukemia have been reported.[10]

Previous dose-finding phase I studies demonstrated that the maximum cumulative administrable activity per cycle of $^{90}$Y-octreotide, with renal protection, is 5.18 GBq.[50] Dosimetric studies showed the advantage of hyperfractionation in lowering the renal and bone marrow dose.[38,46]

Although predicted absorbed doses are lower than the conventional threshold for toxicity, the other target organ raising concerns about acute and permanent toxicity is the bone marrow, particularly in repeated administrations.[3,10,31] The fast pharmacokinetics of radiopeptides, as well as the lack of an evident red marrow uptake in scintigraphic images, indicate a low marrow irradiation. Nonetheless, many effects observed after PRRT were not expected to occur at the low marrow doses estimated (usually <2 Gy, cumulatively). In order to check for additional causes of bone marrow irradiation, the expression of somatostatin receptors on stem cells was postulated. A comparison of the radioactivity concentration in blood and bone marrow aspirates in patients treated with $^{177}$Lu-DOTATATE was performed and linked to the change in platelet counts. The results showed an identical activity concentration in bone marrow and blood and that the radiopharmaceutical does not bind significantly to bone marrow precursor stem cells. No correlation emerged between marrow doses and change in platelet count, and the study confirmed the appropriateness of the models used.[51]

Recently, the study of the possible uptake of $^{111}$In-octreotide and $^{86}$Y-DOTATOC in the bone marrow showed (in single-photon emission CT and PET images collected 24 hours after injection) a faint (~1%) uptake in the spine of some patients, which was not visible in long bones and vertebrae, thus, indicating a receptor-independent of uptake.[52] The study of the in vitro behavior of $^{111}$In-octreotide and $^{86}$Y-DOTATOC, on the other hand, showed a transchelation of $^{111}$In and $^{86}$Y to the free transferrin that could explain the delayed red marrow uptake and, therefore, the toxicity.

As a further source of red marrow irradiation, the possible coexistence of unconjugated radionuclides, such as free $^{90}$Y, which has bone tropism, must be taken into account. This coexistence can occur because of incomplete labeling, impurities, or in vivo deconjugation, as has been reported in relation to several radionuclide therapies.

Finally, the detailed exploration of the acute hematologic events arising after PRRT, with respect to the common severe lymphocytic toxicity, led to the observation that only the B lymphocytes were significantly affected; this explains the benign significance of this occurrence and the absence of secondary infections.[53]

## Others

Finally, the possibility of exacerbation of endocrine symptoms, such as carcinoid, hypoglycemic, or Zollinger-Ellison syndrome, although quite rare, must be carefully considered in syndromic patients. This exacerbation seems to be related to the massive cell lysis and hormonal stimulation occurring after PRRT, which must be prevented and treated accordingly.[54,55]

## EFFICACY

In 17 years of clinical applications, PRRT with [90]Y-octreotide proved to be efficient, with tumor responses, symptom relief, quality-of-life improvement, biomarker reduction, and, ultimately, an impact on survival. **Fig. 1** reports an example of a long-lasting objective response in a patient affected by a G2 pancreatic NET with synchronous liver metastases.

[90]Y-octreotide has been the most-used radiopeptide in the first 8 to 10 years of experience. However, all the published results derive from different phase I and II studies performed independently by various centers and, therefore, inhomogeneous as to the inclusion criteria and treatment schemes. Hence, a direct comparison is virtually impossible to date. Nevertheless, even with these limitations, objective responses are registered in 10% to 34% of patients (**Table 2**).[10,11,31,35–37,39,56–58]

Presently, therapy administration protocols schedule the injection of standard activities that are established from previous escalation studies as well as from clinical experience. This practice results in huge differences among protocols with regard to activities, which may be fixed or related to body weight or surface; number of cycles; and time intervals between cycles.

The first studies with [90]Y-DOTATOC were carried out in relatively advanced phases of disease. The efficacy shown even in these extreme situations led to further trials whereby PRRT was performed in earlier phases of disease with a higher efficacy. This occurence is supported by numerous reasons: primarily radiobiological, related to the volume of tumor masses, and biologic factors because more advanced tumors express less somatostatin receptors and bear many genetic mutations, such as p53, which make them less prone to respond to any treatment. Previous studies have indicated that the tumor load, especially in the liver, and the performance status would influence the outcome of PRRT. Therefore, early treatment rather than a wait-and-see approach is considered to be more advantageous. In addition, the type of disease has to be taken into account because lesions from pancreatic NETs tend to show tumor reduction more frequently compared with other types of NETs.

In a study carried out at Basel University, 39 patients with neuroendocrine tumors, mostly of gastroenteropancreatic origin, were treated with 4 cycles of [90]Y-octreotide, with a cumulative activity of 7.4 GBq. Objective responses, according to the WHO's criteria, were described in 23%, with a complete remission in 2 patients, partial in 7, and a disease stabilization in 27. Pancreatic neuroendocrine tumors (13 patients) showed a better objective response (38% partial + complete) than the other classes did. A significant amelioration of related symptoms occurred in most of the patients.[37]

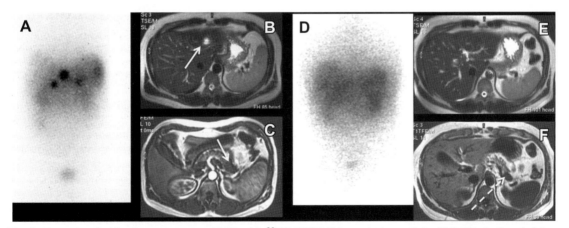

**Fig. 1.** Example of objective response to PRRT with [90]Y-DOTATOC (cumulative activity 12.3 GBq in 5 cycles) in a patient affected by a G2 pancreatic NET with synchronous liver metastases. Basal Octreoscan (*A*) and magnetic resonance (MR) imaging (*B, C*) show the primary tumor in the tail of the pancreas (*C: solid arrow*) and lesions in the left liver lobe (*A, B: solid arrow*). Restaging after completion of PRRT with Octreoscan (*D*) and MR imaging (*E, F: dashed arrow*) shows the disappearance of liver metastases and the persistence of the primary pancreatic lesion. The patient subsequently underwent a splenopancreasectomy with complete eradication of the disease and a long period of absence of any evidence of disease (Time To Progression [TTP] 72 months).

**Table 2**
**Clinical results of PRRT with $^{90}$Y-DOTATOC in NETs**

| Center | Patient Number | CR + PR (%) | Response Criteria | Outcome |
|---|---|---|---|---|
| Basel | 16 | 6 | Nonspecified | Not assessed |
| Milan | 23 | 13 | WHO | Not assessed |
| Basel | 37 | 27 | WHO | TTP>26 mo |
| Basel | 36 | 34 | WHO | Not assessed |
| Milan | 21 | 29 | WHO | TTP 10 mo |
| Multicenter | 58 | 9 | SWOG | TTP 29 mo |
| Warsaw[a] | 58 | 23 | WHO | PFS 17 mo |
| Multicenter | 90 | 4 | SWOG | PFS 16 mo |
| Copenhagen | 53 | 23 | WHO | PFS 29 mo |

*Abbreviations:* CR, complete response; PFS, progression free survival; PR, partial response; SWOG, Southwest Oncology Group; TTP, time to progression; WHO, World Health Organization.
[a] $^{90}$Y-DOTATATE.
*Data from* Refs.[6,35–37,39,50,56–58]

In another multicentric phase I study, carried out at Rotterdam, Louvain, and Tampa Universities, 60 patients affected by gastroenteropancreatic neuroendocrine tumors were treated with 4 cycles of 0.9, 1.8, 2.8, 3.7, 4.6, and 5.5 GBq/m$^2$ administered 6 to 9 weeks apart. In an initial evaluation of the results, published in 2002, in 32 evaluable patients, the objective responses (according to the Southwest Oncology Group [SWOG's] criteria) consisted in about 9% of partial responses and 9% of minor responses.[59] In a later analysis of the same population, published in 2006, on 58 assessable patients who were treated with cumulative activities of 1.7 to 32.8 GBq, a 57% clinical benefit, including stabilization and minor responses, was observed, according to the SWOG's criteria. A true objective response was described in 5% of the patients. The most relevant finding of the study was the observed overall survival, with a median value of about 37 months and a median progression-free survival of about 29 months. These results compared well with the 12-month overall survival of the historical group treated with $^{111}$In-pentetreotide. The median progression-free survival was 29 months.[56]

The results of 2 phase I and II studies and a retrospective evaluation in 141 patients were published by the Milano group in 2004. Patients were affected mainly by neuroendocrine tumors and were treated with a cumulative activity of 7.4 to 26.4 GBq of $^{90}$Y-octreotide, divided into 2 to 16 cycles, administered 4 to 6 weeks apart. The objective response rate was 26%, including partial and complete responses, according to the SWOG's criteria. Disease stabilization was observed in 55% of the patients, and disease progression in 18%. The mean duration of response ranged between 2 and 59 months (median 18). Most of the patients who responded had gastroenteropancreatic neuroendocrine tumors. The study showed that, by dividing the objective response according to the basal status, stable patients at baseline had better outcomes (partial and complete responses in 32%) than did the progressive ones (partial and complete responses in 24%).[31]

Recently, a multicenter study aimed at studying the role of $^{90}$Y-octreotide in 90 patients with symptomatic, metastatic carcinoids, namely, neuroendocrine tumors originating from the small intestines, was published. This study showed that PRRT with $^{90}$Y-octreotide induced the stabilization or tumor response, according to the SWOG's criteria, in 74% of patients as well as a durable amelioration of all the symptoms related to the tumor mass and the hypersecretion of bioactive amines. The symptomatic response had an impact on survival because progression-free survival was significantly longer in those who had durable diarrhea improvement.[58]

More recently, the Basel group published the results of their open-label phase II trial in 1109 patients treated with $^{90}$Y-octreotide, divided in multiple cycles of 3.7 GBq/m$^2$ each. Objective morphologic responses, according to response evaluation criteria in solid tumors (RECIST's) criteria, were observed in 378 (34.1%), biochemical responses in 172 (15.5%), and symptomatic responses in 329 (29.7%). Longer survival was correlated with tumor and symptomatic response. The best predictor of survival was the tumor uptake at baseline.[11]

Protocols combining $^{177}$Lu- and $^{90}$Y-peptides have been recently contemplated in order to benefit from the different physical properties of the radionuclides, although $^{177}$Lu and $^{90}$Y activities have been designed empirically and not on dosimetric values.[22,60]

Regarding the survival after $^{90}$Y-DOTATOC, a phase I–II study on 58 patients with GEP NETs treated with 1.7 to 32.8 GBq reported a clinical benefit (including stabilization and minor response) in 57% (with true objective response in 20%), a median overall survival of 36.7 months (vs 12 months in the historic group treated with $^{111}$In-octreotide), and a median progression-free survival of 29 months. Characteristically, patients stable at baseline had a better overall survival than patients progressive at baseline, and the extent of disease at baseline was a predictive factor for survival.[56]

The American multicentric study published by Bushnell in 2010 in 90 patients showed a progression-free survival of 16 months and an overall survival of 27 months.[58]

The series of 53 Danish patients treated at Basel University showed, comparably, a progression-free survival of 29 months.[36]

Finally, PRRT has also been administered in children and young adults with somatostatin-receptor– positive tumors. A prospective phase I study involved 17 patients (aged 2–24 years) affected by neuroblastomas, MEN2b, gliomas, and neuroendocrine tumors. Patients were treated with $^{90}$Y-octreotide with activities ranging from 1.1 to 1.85 GBq/m$^2$ per cycle for a total of 3 cycles, administered 6 weeks apart. According to the Pediatric Oncology Group's criteria, 12% of partial responses and 29% of minor responses were observed. Improved quality of life during the treatment was a major advantage of the therapy. Therefore, PRRT proved to be efficient and also tolerated in young patients.[61]

Experiences have also been carried out with $^{90}$Y-DOTATATE. A group of 60 patients with histologically proven GEP-NETs were treated with 4.1 to 16.2 GBq per patient (mean 3.7 GBq per therapy) in 1 to 3 cycles. Six months after PRRT completion, PR was registered in 13 patients (23%), whereas the remaining patients showed stable disease (77%). The median progression-free survival was 17 months, whereas the median overall survival was 22 months. Hematological toxicity, WHO grade 3 and 4, was noted during therapy in 10% of patients and persisted in 5%. After 24 months of follow-up, renal toxicity grade 2 was seen in 7 patients; the investigators pointed out the need for a careful renal monitoring.[57]

## FINAL CONSIDERATIONS

PRRT with $^{90}$Y-octreotide demonstrated to be efficient and relatively safe up to the known thresholds of absorbed dose and BED. The toxicity profile is acceptable from a renal and hematological point of view, if necessary protective measures are taken, such as amino acid protection and activity fractionation.

PRRT proved to induce a significant improvement of the quality of life and of all the symptoms related to the disease in most of the treated patients.

Following the pivotal observation of the prognostic value of PET with $^{18}$FDG (Fluoro-Deoxy-Glucose) in predicting the response and progression-free survival after PRRT with $^{177}$Lu-DOTATATE, it is likely that this characteristic can be applied to PRRT with $^{90}$Y-DOTATOC, therefore, indicating the subcategory of FDG-positive patients who might benefit from a more intensive therapeutic approach.[62]

A major open issue remains the definition of the optimal radiopeptide and, even before that, which of the 2 experimented radionuclides is optimal. Even in the absence of randomized trials, some considerations can be made. From the analysis of the residence times for DOTATATE and DOTATOC in the kidneys, $^{177}$Lu seems more beneficial when labeling DOTATATE, whereas, in view of the higher renal dose, $^{90}$Y seems more convenient to label DOTATOC.[9,41] Therefore, from dosimetric projections, the doses to the tumor and normal organs, mainly the kidneys, which result from DOTATATE labeled with $^{90}$Y may increase by a factor of 2 to 4 as compared with $^{177}$Lu. As a result, the benefit/risk balance remains to be established for each patient.[38]

Hence, from a dosimetric point of view, $^{177}$Lu-DOTATATE seems handier than $^{90}$Y-DOTATOC regarding renal and bone marrow doses. However, $^{90}$Y-DOTATOC is more powerful than $^{177}$Lu-DOTATATE regarding the tumor dose. The choice of the radiopeptide depends on the particular clinical scenario of the patient. Bigger lesions may benefit from $^{90}$Y-DOTATOC, whereas smaller ones may benefit from $^{177}$Lu-DOTATATE. Especially when using $^{90}$Y-DOTATOC, particular attention has to be paid to risk factors for renal toxicity, which should suggest caution (lower doses, hyperfractionation) or switching to $^{177}$Lu-DOTATATE.

Results obtained with $^{90}$Y-DOTATOC have been inferred from many phase I–II studies, carried out by various groups, but rather poor in patient number and inhomogeneous as to patient selection, inclusion criteria, and treatment schemes.[12] Therefore, an interstudy comparison is virtually impossible today. Clinical pathology-oriented phase II and phase III trials have been skipped; today the use of PRRT has become quite customary, following enthusiastically the numerous brilliant results obtained in patients. The lack of data still remains, especially on timing and fractionation; but an oncologically correct sequence of clinical trials does not seem feasible anymore for many reasons, logistical, economical, and political. It is hoped that incoming registration phase III clinical studies will help clarify the open issues.

Furthermore, almost all the studies carried out to date focused merely on antitumor activity and, unfortunately, because of the small numbers and relatively short follow-up, still cannot demonstrate with formal oncological significance the impact of PRRT on the most important aim in oncology, namely, the overall survival or at least its surrogate end points, progression-free survival or time to progression.

Finally, patients who are going to respond to PRRT and their specific biologic parameters, such as Ki-67 proliferation index or other individual factors, besides disease extension and basal uptake at receptor imaging, need to be identified.

In addition, the possible renal and bone marrow toxicity is still not fully explored and remains a reason for concern to clinicians, particularly the referring oncologists. Radiation burden to tumor and normal organs, in fact, is difficult to establish with satisfactory accuracy. Nevertheless, treating patients with an excessively conservative approach, not considering the individual dosimetry, may limit in turn the efficacy of treatment.

Unfortunately, the search for efficacy is not independent from the possibility of toxicity; the treatment of neuroendocrine tumors with PRRT has been rightfully compared with the journey of Ulysses, trying to steer a course between the 2 sea monsters, on one side Scylla, who, like a tumor, ate sailors with his multiple heads and jaws, and, on the other side, Charybdis, who, like toxicity, devoured ships with his whirlpools.[50]

In this regard, the comprehension of the radiobiologic and of individual, genetically based features inherent to radiopeptide therapy could allow a patient-tailored treatment, with the most efficient tumor irradiation and, at the same time, the most conservative safety profile with respect to normal organs.

# REFERENCES

1. Zaknun JJ, Bodei L, Mueller-Brand J, et al. The joint IAEA, EANM, and SNMMI practical guidance on peptide receptor radionuclide therapy (PRRNT) in neuroendocrine tumours. Eur J Nucl Med Mol Imaging 2013;40(5):800–16.
2. Krenning EP, Kooij PP, Bakker WH, et al. Radiotherapy with a radiolabeled somatostatin analogue, [111In-DTPA-D-Phe1]-octreotide. A case history. Ann N Y Acad Sci 1994;733:496–506.
3. Valkema R, De Jong M, Bakker WH, et al. Phase I study of peptide receptor radionuclide therapy with [In-DTPA]-octreotide: the Rotterdam experience. Semin Nucl Med 2002;32(2):110–22.
4. Heppeler A, Froidevaux S, Maecke HR, et al. Radiometal-labelled macrocyclic chelator-derivatised somatostatin analogue with superb tumour-targeting properties and potential for receptor-mediated internal radiotherapy. Chem Eur J 1999;7:1974–81.
5. de Jong M, Bakker WH, Krenning EP, et al. Yttrium-90 and indium-111 labelling, receptor binding and biodistribution of [DOTA0, d-Phe1, Tyr3] octreotide, a promising somatostatin analogue for radionuclide therapy. Eur J Nucl Med 1997;24(4):368–71.
6. Otte A, Mueller-Brand J, Dellas S, et al. Yttrium-90-labelled somatostatin-analogue for cancer treatment. Lancet 1998;351(9100):417–8.
7. Virgolini I, Britton K, Buscombe J, et al. In- and Y-DOTA-lanreotide: results and implications of the MAURITIUS trial. Semin Nucl Med 2002;32(2):148–55.
8. Kwekkeboom DJ, Bakker WH, Kooij PP, et al. [177Lu-DOTA0Tyr3] octreotate: comparison with [111In-DTPA0] octreotide in patients. Eur J Nucl Med 2001;28(9):1319–25.
9. Bodei L, Ferone D, Grana CM, et al. Peptide receptor therapies in neuroendocrine tumors. J Endocrinol Invest 2009;32(4):360–9.
10. Kwekkeboom DJ, Mueller-Brand J, Paganelli G, et al. Overview of results of peptide receptor radionuclide therapy with 3 radiolabeled somatostatin analogs. J Nucl Med 2005;46(Suppl 1):62S–6S.
11. Imhof A, Brunner P, Marincek N, et al. Response, survival, and long-term toxicity after therapy with the radiolabeled somatostatin analogue [90Y-DOTA]-TOC in metastasized neuroendocrine cancers. J Clin Oncol 2011;29(17):2416–23.
12. Kwekkeboom DJ, Kam BL, van Essen M, et al. Somatostatin-receptor-based imaging and therapy of gastroenteropancreatic neuroendocrine tumors. Endocr Relat Cancer 2010;17(1):R53–73.
13. Pauwels S, Barone R, Walrand S, et al. Practical dosimetry of peptide receptor radionuclide therapy with (90)Y-labeled somatostatin analogs. J Nucl Med 2005;46(Suppl 1):92S–8S.
14. Focosi D, Cecconi N, Boni G, et al. Acute myeloid leukaemia after treatment with (90)Y-ibritumomab tiuxetan for follicular lymphoma. Hematol Oncol 2008;26(3):179–81.
15. Dale R, Carabe-Fernandez A. The radiobiology of conventional radiotherapy and its application to radionuclide therapy. Cancer Biother Radiopharm 2005;20(1):47–51.
16. Dale R. Use of the linear-quadratic radiobiological model for quantifying kidney response in targeted

radiotherapy. Cancer Biother Radiopharm 2004; 19(3):363–70.

17. Barone R, Borson-Chazot F, Valkema R, et al. Patient-specific dosimetry in predicting renal toxicity with (90)Y-DOTATOC: relevance of kidney volume and dose rate in finding a dose–effect relationship. J Nucl Med 2005;46(Suppl 1):99S–106S.

18. Parliament MB, Murray D. Single nucleotide polymorphisms of DNA repair genes as predictors of radioresponse. Semin Radiat Oncol 2010;20(4): 232–40.

19. Wilson GD. Cell kinetics. Clin Oncol (R Coll Radiol) 2007;19(6):370–84.

20. Konijnenberg MW, de Jong M. Preclinical animal research on therapy dosimetry with dual isotopes. Eur J Nucl Med Mol Imaging 2011;38(Suppl 1): S19–27.

21. Brans B, Bodei L, Giammarile F, et al. Clinical radionuclide therapy dosimetry: the quest for the "Holy Gray". Eur J Nucl Med Mol Imaging 2007; 34(5):772–86.

22. de Jong M, Breeman WA, Valkema R, et al. Combination radionuclide therapy using 177Lu- and 90Y-labeled somatostatin analogs. J Nucl Med 2005;46: 13S–7S.

23. Garkavij M, Nickel M, Sjögreen-Gleisner K, et al. 177Lu-[DOTA0, Tyr3] octreotate therapy in patients with disseminated neuroendocrine tumors: analysis of dosimetry with impact on future therapeutic strategy. Cancer 2010;116(Suppl 4): 1084–92.

24. van Essen M, Krenning EP, Kam BL, et al. Salvage therapy with (177)Lu-octreotate in patients with bronchial and gastroenteropancreatic neuroendocrine tumors. J Nucl Med 2010;51(3):383–90.

25. Guerriero F, Ferrari ME, Botta F, et al. Kidney dosimetry in (177)Lu and (90)y peptide receptor radionuclide therapy: influence of image timing, time-activity integration method, and risk factors. Biomed Res Int 2013;2013:935351. http://dx.doi.org/10.1155/2013/935351.

26. Larsson M, Bernhardt P, Svensson JB, et al. Estimation of absorbed dose to the kidneys in patients after treatment with 177Lu-octreotate: comparison between methods based on planar scintigraphy. EJNMMI Res 2012;2(1):49.

27. Sandström M, Garske U, Granberg D, et al. Individualized dosimetry in patients undergoing therapy with (177)Lu-DOTA-D-Phe (1)-Tyr (3)-octreotate. Eur J Nucl Med Mol Imaging 2010;37(2):212–25.

28. Cremonesi M, Ferrari M, Bodei L, et al. Dosimetry in peptide radionuclide receptor therapy: a review. J Nucl Med 2006;47(9):1467–75.

29. Walrand S, Jamar F, Mathieu I, et al. Quantitation in PET using isotopes emitting prompt single gammas: application to yttrium-86. Eur J Nucl Med Mol Imaging 2003;30(3):354–61.

30. Reubi JC, Schär JC, Waser B, et al. Affinity profiles for human somatostatin receptor subtypes SST1-SST5 of somatostatin radiotracers selected for scintigraphic and radiotherapeutic use. Eur J Nucl Med 2000;27(3):273–82.

31. Bodei L, Cremonesi M, Grana C, et al. Receptor radionuclide therapy with 90Y-[DOTA]0-Tyr3-octreotide (90Y-DOTATOC) in neuroendocrine tumours. Eur J Nucl Med Mol Imaging 2004;31(7): 1038–46.

32. Jamar F, Barone R, Mathieu I, et al. (86Y-DOTA0)-D-Phe1-Tyr3-octreotide (SMT487)–a phase 1 clinical study: pharmacokinetics, biodistribution and renal protective effect of different regimens of amino acid co-infusion. Eur J Nucl Med Mol Imaging 2003;30(4):510–8.

33. Minarik D, Ljungberg M, Segars P, et al. Evaluation of quantitative planar 90Y bremsstrahlung whole-body imaging. Phys Med Biol 2009;54(19): 5873–83.

34. Walrand S, Flux GD, Konijnenberg MW, et al. Dosimetry of yttrium-labelled radiopharmaceuticals for internal therapy: 86Y or 90Y imaging? Eur J Nucl Med Mol Imaging 2011;38(Suppl 1):S57–68.

35. Waldherr C, Pless M, Maecke HR, et al. The clinical value of [90Y-DOTA]-D-Phe1-Tyr3-octreotide (90Y-DOTATOC) in the treatment of neuroendocrine tumours: a clinical phase II study. Ann Oncol 2001; 12:941–5.

36. Pfeifer AK, Gregersen T, Gronbaek H, et al. Peptide receptor radionuclide therapy with Y-DOTA-TOC and (177)Lu-DOTATOC in advanced neuroendocrine tumors: results from a Danish cohort treated in Switzerland. Neuroendocrinology 2011;93:189–96.

37. Waldherr C, Pless M, Maecke HR, et al. Tumor response and clinical benefit in neuroendocrine tumors after 7.4 GBq (90)Y-DOTATOC. J Nucl Med 2002;43(5):610–6.

38. Cremonesi M, Botta F, Di Dia A, et al. Dosimetry for treatment with radiolabelled somatostatin analogues. A review. Q J Nucl Med Mol Imaging 2010;54(1):37–51.

39. Paganelli G, Zoboli S, Cremonesi M, et al. Receptor-mediated radiotherapy with 90Y-DOTA-D-Phe1–Tyr3-octreotide. Eur J Nucl Med 2001;28: 426–34.

40. Cassady JR. Clinical radiation nephropathy. Int J Radiat Oncol Biol Phys 1995;31(5):1249–56.

41. Esser JP, Krenning EP, Teunissen JJ, et al. Comparison of [(177)Lu-DOTA(0), Tyr(3)]octreotate and [(177)Lu-DOTA(0), Tyr(3)]octreotide: which peptide is preferable for PRRT? Eur J Nucl Med Mol Imaging 2006;33(11):1346–51.

42. de Jong M, Krenning EP. New advances in peptide receptor radionuclide therapy. J Nucl Med 2002; 43(5):617–20.

43. Bernard BF, Krenning EP, Breeman WA, et al. D-lysine reduction of indium-111 octreotide and yttrium-90 octreotide renal uptake. J Nucl Med 1997;38(12):1929–33.

44. Valkema R, Pauwels SA, Kvols LK, et al. Long-term follow-up of renal function after peptide receptor radiation therapy with (90)Y-DOTA(0), Tyr(3)- octreotide and (177)Lu-DOTA(0), Tyr(3)-octreotate. J Nucl Med 2005;46(Suppl 1):83S–91S.

45. Cybulla M, Weiner SM, Otte A. End-stage renal disease after treatment with 90Y-DOTATOC. Eur J Nucl Med 2001;28(10):1552–4.

46. Bodei L, Cremonesi M, Ferrari M, et al. Long-term evaluation of renal toxicity after peptide receptor radionuclide therapy with 90Y-DOTATOC and 177Lu-DOTATATE: the role of associated risk factors. Eur J Nucl Med Mol Imaging 2008;35(10): 1847–56.

47. Konijnenberg MW, Bijster M, Krenning EP, et al. A stylized computational model of the rat for organ dosimetry in support of preclinical evaluations of peptide receptor radionuclide therapy with (90)Y, (111)In, or (177)Lu. J Nucl Med 2004;45(7): 1260–9 [Erratum appears in J Nucl Med 2009; 50(12):2092].

48. Konijnenberg M, Melis M, Valkema R, et al. Radiation dose distribution in human kidneys by octreotides in peptide receptor radionuclide therapy. J Nucl Med 2007;48(1):134–42.

49. Nicolas G, Campana B, Forrer F. Ex-vivo autoradiographic study registered with histopathological sections demonstrates inhomogeneous radioactivity distribution after therapeutic application of $^{90}Y/^{111}In$-DOTATOC. Eur J Nucl Med Mol Imaging 2010;37(S2):S368.P179.

50. Bodei L, Cremonesi M, Zoboli S, et al. Receptor-mediated radionuclide therapy with 90Y-DOTATOC in association with amino acid infusion: a phase I study. Eur J Nucl Med Mol Imaging 2003;30(2): 207–16.

51. Forrer F, Krenning EP, Kooij PP, et al. Bone marrow dosimetry in peptide receptor radionuclide therapy with [177Lu-DOTA(0), Tyr(3)] octreotate. Eur J Nucl Med Mol Imaging 2009;36(7):1138–46.

52. Walrand S, Barone R, Pauwels S, et al. Experimental facts supporting a red marrow uptake due to radiometal transchelation in 90Y-DOTATOC therapy and relationship to the decrease of platelet counts. Eur J Nucl Med Mol Imaging 2011;38(7): 1270–80.

53. Sierra ML, Agazzi A, Bodei L, et al. Lymphocytic toxicity in patients after peptide-receptor radionuclide therapy (PRRT) with 177Lu-DOTATATE and 90Y-DOTATOC. Cancer Biother Radiopharm 2009; 24(6):659–65.

54. Davì MV, Bodei L, Francia G, et al. Carcinoid crisis induced by receptor radionuclide therapy with 90Y-DOTATOC in a case of liver metastases from bronchial neuroendocrine tumor (atypical carcinoid). J Endocrinol Invest 2006;29(6):563–7.

55. de Keizer B, van Aken MO, Feelders RA, et al. Hormonal crises following receptor radionuclide therapy with the radiolabeled somatostatin analogue [177Lu-DOTA0, Tyr3] octreotide. Eur J Nucl Med Mol Imaging 2008;35(4):749–55.

56. Valkema R, Pauwels S, Kvols LK, et al. Survival and response after peptide receptor radionuclide therapy with [90Y-DOTA0, Tyr3]octreotide in patients with advanced gastroenteropancreatic neuroendocrine tumors. Semin Nucl Med 2006; 36(2):147–56.

57. Cwikla JB, Sankowski A, Seklecka N, et al. Efficacy of radionuclide treatment DOTATATE Y-90 in patients with progressive metastatic gastroenteropancreatic neuroendocrine carcinomas (GEP-NETs): a phase II study. Ann Oncol 2010; 21:787–94.

58. Bushnell DL Jr, O'Dorisio TM, O'Dorisio MS, et al. 90Y-edotreotide for metastatic carcinoid refractory to octreotide. J Clin Oncol 2010;28(10):1652–9.

59. De Jong M, Valkema R, Jamar F, et al. Somatostatin receptor-targeted radionuclide therapy of tumors: preclinical and clinical findings. Semin Nucl Med 2002;32(2):133–40.

60. Kunikowska J, Królicki L, Hubalewska-Dydejczyk A, et al. Clinical results of radionuclide therapy of neuroendocrine tumours with (90)Y-DOTATATE and tandem (90)Y/(177)Lu-DOTATATE: which is a better therapy option? Eur J Nucl Med Mol Imaging 2011;38(10):1788–97.

61. Menda Y, O'Dorisio MS, Kao S, et al. Phase I trial of 90Y-DOTATOC therapy in children and young adults with refractory solid tumors that express somatostatin receptors. J Nucl Med 2010;51(10): 1524–31.

62. Severi S, Nanni O, Bodei L, et al. Role of 18FDG PET/CT in patients treated with 177Lu-DOTATATE for advanced differentiated neuroendocrine tumours. Eur J Nucl Med Mol Imaging 2013;40(6): 881–8.

# Section II: Theranostics of Neuroendocrine Neoplasms

# Patient Selection for Personalized Peptide Receptor Radionuclide Therapy Using Ga-68 Somatostatin Receptor PET/CT

Harshad R. Kulkarni, MD*, Richard P. Baum, MD, PhD

## KEYWORDS

- Ga-68 • PRRT • Somatostatin receptors

## KEY POINTS

- Neuroendocrine tumors (NETs) are malignant solid tumors originating from neuroendocrine cells dispersed throughout the body.
- Differentiated NETs overexpress somatostatin receptors (SSTRs), which enable the diagnosis using radiolabeled somatostatin analogues.
- Internalization and retention within the tumor cell are important for peptide receptor radionuclide therapy (PRRT). Use of the same DOTA peptide for SSTR PET/CT using [68]Ga and for PRRT using therapeutic radionuclides like [177]Lu and [90]Y offers a unique theranostic advantage.
- This forms the basis for the role of [68]Ga-SSTR PET/CT not only in patient selection for PRRT but also for prognostication, assessment of therapeutic response, and long-term follow-up after PRRT.

## HOW DOES SUV RELATE WITH SSTR DENSITY?

PET imaging enables a semi-quantitative analysis of the tracer uptake with standardized uptake values (SUVs).[1,2] It is independent of the amount of injected activity rather a function of time. Our group (Kaemmerer and colleagues[3]) aimed to clarify if there was a correlation between somatostatin receptor (SSTR) PET/CT, using the SUV as a parameter of the SSTR density in gastroentero-pancreatic (GEP-NETs) and/or its metastases, and the expression intensity of the 5 SSTR subtypes in surgically removed GEP-NET tissue, evaluated by immunohistochemistry (IHC). Therefore, this study aimed to accurately quantify the SSTR distribution of all 5 SSTR subtypes in different

GEP-NETs using IHC. The preoperative [68]Ga-SSTR PET/CT was analyzed in 34 histologically documented GEP-NET patients. A total of 44 surgical specimens were generated. Only lesions greater than 1.5 cm on PET/CT were selected to avoid partial volume effect on the semi-quantitative parameters. The IHC scores for SSTR2A and SSTR5 correlated significantly with the $SUV_{max}$ on the PET/CT, whereas only SSTR2A IHC score correlated significantly with $SUV_{mean}$ and CgA staining as well as inversely with the tumor grade.

Miederer and colleagues[4] compared a score of SSTR2 IHC with the in vivo SUV of preoperative or prebiopsy [68]Ga-DOTATOC PET/CT in 18 patients. They noted that negative IHC scores were

THERANOSTICS Center for Molecular Radiotherapy and Molecular Imaging, ENETS Center of Excellence, Zentralklinik Bad Berka, Robert-Koch-Alle 9, 99437 Bad Berka, Germany
* Corresponding author.
E-mail address: harshad.kulkarni@zentralklinik.de

PET Clin 9 (2014) 83–90
http://dx.doi.org/10.1016/j.cpet.2013.08.015
1556-8598/14/$ – see front matter © 2014 Elsevier Inc. All rights reserved.

consistent with SUV values less than 10 and all specimens with a score of 2 and 3 corresponded with high SUVs (>15). They concluded that because there was a good correlation between SSTR2-IHC scores and SUVs, SSTR2-IHC analysis in patients missing a preoperative PET scan could indicate [68]Ga-DOTATOC-PET/CT as method for restaging and follow-up in individual patients. Müssig and colleagues[5] also showed the association of SSTR 2 immunohistochemical expression with [111]In-DTPA octreotide scintigraphy and [68]Ga-DOTATOC PET/CT in NETs. Boy and colleagues[6] measured the [68]Ga-DOTATOC $SUV_{max}$ of normal tissues in 120 patients. Expression of SSTR subtypes 1 to 5 was measured independently in pooled adult normal human tissue by real-time reverse transcriptase polymerase chain reaction. $SUV_{max}$ values exclusively correlated with SSTR 2 expression at the level of mRNA.

## IMPACT OF [68]GA-SSTR PET/CT ON MANAGEMENT OF NETS

Peptide receptor radionuclide therapy (PRRT) is an effective treatment option for metastasized progressive well-differentiated NETs[1]. [68]Ga-SSTR PET/CT provides in vivo histopathology by quantification of the SSTR expression (receptor density) in NETs by the SUV measurement.[3] Thus the way to personalized medicine starts with tissue sampling followed by histopathological analysis, which should consist of grading (ie, based on proliferation rate Ki-67/MIB 1 index), staining for chromogranin A, and synaptophysin, and quantification of the SSTR density on tumor cells. Based on these data, the most appropriate peptide (DOTA-TOC/TATE, broad spectrum agonist, or an antagonist) can be selected for SSTR PET/CT. The theranostic advantage of using the same peptide allows for patient selection and also to predict the effectiveness of PRRT (depending on the strength of uptake) (**Figs. 1** and **2**). The determination of size on CT and MRI alone is not reliable enough because of the possibility of cystic degeneration of metastases. In addition, assessment of the tumor burden (localized disease vs distant metastases) by SSTR PET/CT guides the therapeutic options. For example, localized, bulky liver metastases can be effectively managed by intra-arterial PRRT, although partial hepatectomy and hepatic transplantation are also options. The amount of radioactivity to be administered as well as the

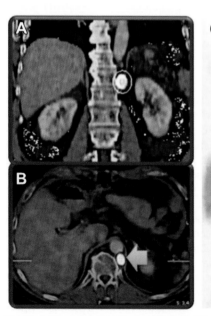
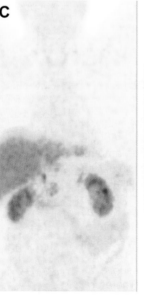
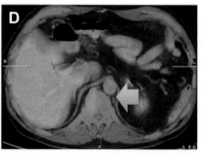

Fig. 1. A 66-year-old patient with well-differentiated, nonfunctioning NET of the pancreas, status post left pancreatectomy, splenectomy, and also metastasectomy in segment 2 of the liver was referred for follow-up [68]Ga-SSTR PET/CT after surgery, which revealed a single, very intensely SSTR-positive retrocrural lymph node metastasis with an SUV of 152. Based on this, he underwent 2 cycles of PRRT with 14 GBq [177]Lu-DOTATATE. The very high receptor expression and uptake of [177]Lu and the resulting high dose delivered to the metastasis resulted in a complete remission according to molecular response criteria, after the 2 PRRT cycles. (*A*) Fused coronal [68]Ga-DOTATATE PET/CT before therapy and (*B*) fused transverse image before therapy showing the lymph node metastasis with a *circle* and *arrow*, respectively. (*C*) MIP image of [68]Ga-DOTATATE PET/CT after 2 therapy cycles and (*D*) corresponding fused transverse posttherapy image confirmed molecular complete remission, although a small lymph node (*arrow*) is still noted on the CT, which remained stable in size over the next years of follow-up.

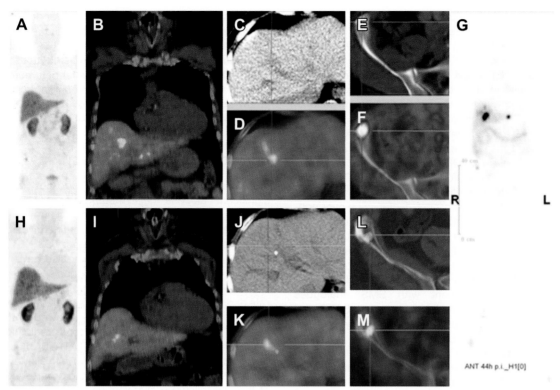

Fig. 2. A 56-year-old man with well-differentiated, nonfunctioning ileal NET status post surgery and 2 cycles of PRRT with $^{90}$Y-DOTATOC (performed elsewhere) with complete remission of the hepatic metastases thereafter was referred to the authors' center 5 years after the second PRRT cycle with progressive disease and development of hepatic and osseous metastases. He underwent 2 further cycles of PRRT with a total administered activity of 8 GBq $^{177}$Lu-DOTATATE, resulting in a good response of the hepatic metastases (near-complete remission) and of the lesion in right iliac bone (partial remission). (A–F, $^{68}$Ga-DOTATATE PET/CT images before therapy; G, $^{177}$Lu-DO-TATATE whole-body planar scan 44 hours post-PRRT1; H-M, $^{68}$Ga-DOTATATE PET/CT images after 2 PRRT cycles; A and H, MIP; B and I, fused coronal images; C and J, transverse CT, and D and K, fused transverse PET/CT images of liver; E and L, transverse CT, and F and M, fused transverse PET/CT images showing metastasis in the right ilium).

timing of PRRT using $^{177}$Lu- or $^{90}$Y-DOTATATE or DOTATOC depends on - among other factors - the semi-quantitative interpretation of $^{68}$Ga-SSTR PET/CT.

Curative treatment of localized NETs is possible by complete surgical resection of the primary tumor with accompanying regional lymph node metastases. However, in advanced disease with metastases, palliative therapies can be administered, taking into account the tumor stage, size, localization, and degree of differentiation. The options available apart from PRRT are surgery, somatostatin (SMS) analogues, immunologic therapy (interferon), targeted therapy with kinase inhibitors, radiofrequency ablation, and trans-arterial chemoembolization as well as chemotherapy (in pancreatic NETs and fast-growing grade 3 neuroendocrine carcinomas). Receptor PET/CT also helps in therapy stratification and, for example, excluding PRRT as a therapy option when chemotherapy or molecular therapy in the

case of inadequate receptor expression is indicated for the selection of patients for local therapy (radiofrequency ablation/trans-arterial chemoembolization) of localized liver disease, and so on.

$^{111}$In-octreotide has been considered to be the gold standard for the diagnosis of NETs.[7] However, there are several reasons to think that this method will gradually become the "old" standard because the development of novel SMS analogues for labeling with $^{68}$Ga has revolutionized the diagnostics of NETs by high specific targeting and paved the way to theranostics. A recent meta-analysis showed its patient-wise pooled sensitivity to be 93% and specificity 91%.[8] As early as in 2001, Hofmann and colleagues[9] had demonstrated that $^{68}$Ga-DOTATOC was superior to $^{111}$In-octreotide SPECT in detecting upper abdominal metastases. Similarly for the detection of metastases in lungs, bone, liver, and brain $^{68}$Ga-DOTATOC PET/CT had a clear edge over $^{111}$In-DTPAOC, shown by Buchmann and colleagues.[10] On a per patient basis, [68]Ga-DOTA-TOC PET (96%) was also found to be more accurate than CT (75%) and [111]In-DOTATOC SPECT (58%).[11] Also regarding the sensitivity,[12] [68]Ga-DOTATOC PET fared better than [111]In-octreotide especially in detecting small tumors or tumors bearing only a low density of SSTRs. In patients with equivocal or negative Octreoscan, [68]Ga-DOTATATE PET/CT detected additional lesions and changed management of the disease, notably in 36 patients (70.6%), who were subsequently deemed suitable for PRRT.[13] [68]Ga-DOTANOC PET/CT had a significant impact on the therapeutic management, with incremental value over conventional imaging (CT and EUS), affecting either stage or therapy in 50 of 90 (55.5%) patients.[14] The noteworthy and also the most frequent impact on management was either initiation or continuation of PRRT. SSTR PET could also exclude 2 patients from treatment with SMS analogues because the lesions did not express SSTR and could also avoid unnecessary surgery and the accompanying morbidity in 6 patients.

In pulmonary NETs as well, [68]Ga-DOTATATE was shown to have a definite incremental value over [18]F-FDG for typical bronchial carcinoids and not in atypical carcinoids or higher grades of tumors,[15] Demonstrating the value of SSTR PET/CT for appropriate patient selection for PRRT, namely those with metastatic typical carcinoids. The probability of the presence and/or development of concomitant GEP-NETs should also be borne in mind, which then could be handled in time with PRRT if necessary. SSTR PET/CT with [68]Ga should also therefore be used for the long-term follow-up of pulmonary NETs.[16]

In a bicentric study, the role of [68]Ga DOTANOC PET/CT was found to be highly superior to [111]In-Octreoscan and CT for the detection of an unknown primary (Cancer of unknown Primary [CUP]-NETs).[17] The maximum SUVs of CUP-NETs were also compared with those of known pancreatic NETs and ileal/jejunal/duodenal NETs (small intestinal NETs). Interestingly, the SUV$_{max}$ of the previously unknown pancreatic NETs and small intestinal NETs were significantly lower (P<.05) than SUV$_{max}$ of known primary tumors. Ten percent of the patients were operated based on [68]Ga-SSTR PET/CT, although in most patients, the primary tumors were not operated because of the presence of distant metastases. These patients could be the candidates for PRRT.

An important difference between [68]Ga-SSTR PET/CT and SRS using [111]In-pentetreotide is the quantitative assessment of SSTR density before PRRT, rather than just looking at the images. PET/CT enables accurate determination of the disease burden and quantifies the receptor density on tumor cells. Therefore, the next step after patient selection is the planning of PRRT. Prasad and Baum[18] demonstrated the biodistribution of [68]Ga-DOTANOC in normal tissues and tumors, which revealed a very wide variation (**Table 1**), emphasizing the importance of determining SUVs for an accurate assessment of disease.

## ADDITIONAL ROLE OF FDG PET/CT

Well-differentiated tumors generally do not have significant glucose hypermetabolism. [18]F-FDG PET/CT has a role in metabolically highly active tumors and is recommended as a routine investigation for the diagnosis and staging of G3 NETs (**Fig. 3**). However, [18]F-FDG PET may also have a role in the assessment of prognosis before PRRT. A correlation between the proliferation rate and detection with [18]F-FDG has been demonstrated. Severi and coworkers[19] showed that FDG-PET evaluation is useful for predicting response to PRRT (using [177]Lu-DOTATATE) in patients with grade 1/2 advanced NETs. In this study, none of the PET-negative patients had progressed at the first follow-up examination after PRRT. On the other hand, grade 2 and PET-positive NET (arbitrary SUV cutoff >2.5) were frequently associated with more aggressive disease. Indeed 32% of the PET-positive patients with grade 2 NET did not respond to PRRT monotherapy, which led to the

**Table 1**
**Variation of uptake on [68]Ga-SSTR PET/CT**

| Organ | Range |
| --- | --- |
| Pituitary | 0.8–7.6 |
| Thyroid | 0.6–11.4 |
| Lung | 0.2–1.8 |
| Liver | 4.2–13.4 |
| Spleen | 7.2–48.5 |
| Adrenal | 2.4–13.9 |
| Kidney | 4.1–21.5 |
| Intestine | 0.9–4.3 |
| Gluteal | 0.4–2.2 |
| Femur | 0.4–1.9 |
| Blood pool | 0.8–3.9 |
| Uncinate process of pancreas | 4–9.7 |
| Tumor | 1.6–152 |

*Data from* Prasad V, Baum RP. Biodistribution of the Ga-68 labeled somatostatin analogue DOTA-NOC in patients with neuroendocrine tumors: characterization of uptake in normal organs and tumor lesions. Q J Nucl Med Mol Imaging 2010;54:61–7.

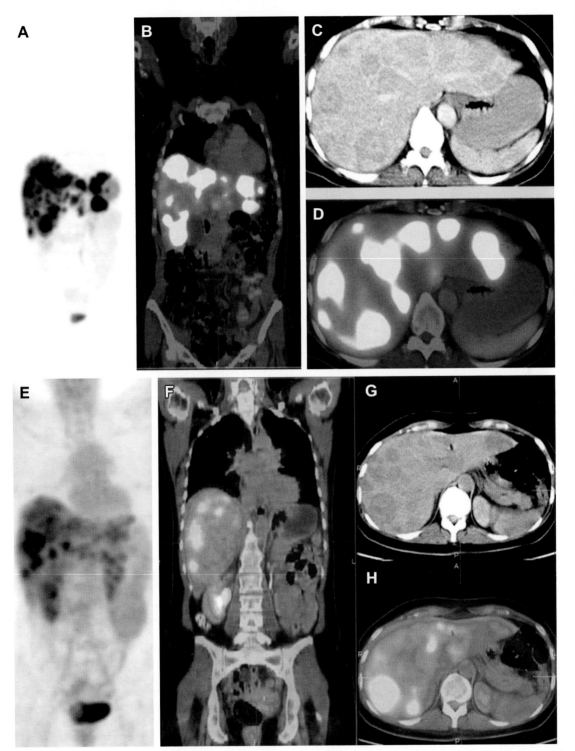

**Fig. 3.** A 45-year-old female patient with a poorly differentiated (G3), nonfunctional neuroendocrine carcinoma of the pancreas with extensive liver metastases. The proliferation rate (Ki-67) of the tumor was 40% with expression of chromogranin A, synaptophysin, and CD 56. She had undergone chemotherapy with Carboplatin and Etoposide, however, with poor results and progressive leucocytopenia. Both $^{68}$Ga-DOTATOC SSTR PET/CT as well as $^{18}$F-FDG PET/CT were performed to assess the option of PRRT and to evaluate the prognosis, respectively. Despite a high grade of the tumor, there was a very high SSTR expression by the disseminated hepatic metastases, with an $SUV_{max}$ of 71.7. No extrahepatic metastases were seen. Notably, $^{18}$F-FDG PET/CT showed a complete matched finding with glucose hypermetabolism of the liver metastases ($SUV_{max}$ of 9.9). With high SSTR expression by the liver metastases, the indication for PRRT was confirmed, which was further demonstrated by the high uptake of $^{177}$Lu-DOTATOC (after the first PRRT cycle) in the metastases. $^{68}$Ga-DOTATOC PET/CT: (*A*) MIP; (*B*) fused coronal PET/CT; (*C*) transverse CT; (*D*) fused transverse PET/CT. $^{18}$F-FDG PET/CT: (*E*) MIP; (*F*) fused coronal PET/CT; (*G*) transverse CT; (*H*) fused transverse PET/CT. $^{177}$Lu-DOTATOC whole-body planar image post-therapy: (*I*) anterior view; (*J*) posterior view.

I        J

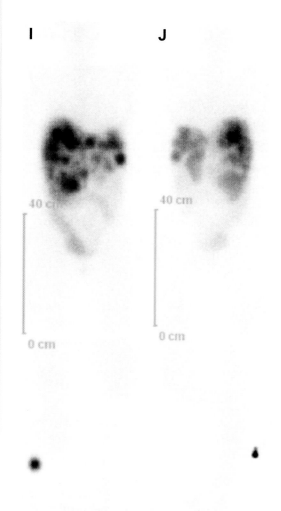

40 cm        40 cm

0 cm        0 cm

**Fig. 3.** (*continued*)

conclusion that these patients might benefit from more intensive therapy protocols, such as the combination of chemotherapy and PRRT.

## PRETHERAPEUTIC SUVS AND POSTTHERAPEUTIC RESPONSE

Pauwels and coauthors[20] assessed tumor dose-response relationship in 13 patients treated with [90]Y-DOTATOC. Tumor volumes were assessed by CT before and after treatment. Tumor dose estimates were derived from CT scan volume measurements and quantitative [86]Y-DOTATOC imaging performed before treatment. A good correlation was found between [86]Y-DOTATOC dosimetry and treatment outcome. Importantly, a tumor size reduction was always seen with a tumor dose of more than 100 Gy, confirming a tumor dose-response relationship in PRRT.

We presented preliminary results also indicating a relationship between the radiation dose delivered to liver metastases and the molecular response post-PRRT as measured by SSTR PET/CT.[21] Ninety-six liver metastases were analyzed in 67 patients with well-differentiated NETs, undergoing PRRT with 4.8 to 7.5 GBq of [177]Lu-DOTA-TOC/-TATE followed by 5 whole-body planar scintigraphies after therapy for dosimetry. Pre- and posttherapy SSTR PET/CT with [68]Ga-DOTA-TOC/-TATE were performed to evaluate molecular response to therapy. Liver metastases were divided into 2 groups based on the response according to molecular imaging criteria: partial response (ie, 15% or more fall in $SUV_{max}$ [group 1]) and progressive disease (ie, 25% or more increase in the $SUV_{max}$ [group 2]). Logarithmic increase in molecular response was observed with increasing mean absorbed dose to tumor. Doses delivered (mean/median) to lesions showing a therapy response (143 Gy/79 Gy) were significantly higher than doses to lesions showing minor progression or progressive disease (23 Gy/20 Gy).

Ezziddin and colleagues[22] investigated the correlation between the pretherapeutic tumor SUV in [68]Ga-SSTR PET/CT using DOTATOC, and the mean absorbed tumor dose during subsequent PRRT using [177]Lu- DOTATATE; this was a retrospective analysis of 21 NET patients with 61 evaluable tumor lesions undergoing both pretherapeutic [68]Ga-DOTATOC-PET/CT and PRRT with [177]Lu-DOTATATE. The SUVs were compared with tumor-absorbed doses per injected activity (D/A0) of the subsequent first treatment cycle. There was a significant correlation between both, $SUV_{mean}$ and $SUV_{max}$ on the one hand, and the D/A0. Pancreatic origin and hepatic localization were associated with higher D/A0. Chromogranin A level and Ki-67 index had no influence on SUV or D/A0, whereas high-SUV lesions resulted in high D/A0. The authors concluded that SSTR PET imaging may predict the mean absorbed tumor doses, and therefore, could aid in selection of appropriate candidates for PRRT. Keeping the dose-response relationship in mind, this study indicates that the pretherapeutic SUVs could predict the response to PRRT. However, a recently published study indicated a poor correlation between SUV and the tumor dose, and the linear regression analysis provided R2 values, which explained only a small fraction of the total variance. It was concluded that the SUVs derived from [68]Ga-SSTR PET/CT images should be used with caution for the prediction of tumor dose on [177]Lu-PRRT, as there was a large intra- and interpatient variability.[23]

The role of [68]Ga-SSTR PET/CT for the evaluation of prognosis of NETs has been investigated.

**Table 2**
**Factors determining the Bad Berka Score for patient selection**

| Factor | Means of Determination |
|---|---|
| Tumor grade | Ki-67 index |
| Functional activity of the tumor/metastases | Biomarkers, symptoms |
| Time since first diagnosis and previous therapies | History |
| General status of the patient | Karnofsky performance score or Eastern Cooperative Oncology Group performance status scale, loss of weight |
| SSTR density | SUV on $^{68}$Ga-receptor PET/CT |
| Glucose metabolism | $^{18}$F-FDG PET/CT |
| Renal functional assessment | Creatinine and blood urea nitrogen |
| Tubular extraction rate and elimination kinetics | $^{99m}$Tc-MAG3 scintigraphy |
| Glomerular filtration rate | $^{99m}$Tc-DTPA |
| Hematological status | Blood counts |
| Hepatic involvement and extrahepatic tumor burden | $^{68}$Ga-receptor PET/CT |
| Dynamics of the disease: doubling time, appearance of new lesions | Serial $^{68}$Ga-receptor PET/CT |

In a study of 47 patients, $SUV_{max}$ was demonstrated to be significantly higher in patients with pancreatic NETs and in those with well-differentiated tumors.[24] On follow-up, stable disease or partial response was observed in 25 patients, and progressive disease in 19 patients. Stable disease or partial response was associated with a significantly higher $SUV_{max}$ than was progressive disease, the best cutoff ranging from 17.9 to 19.3. At univariate and multivariate analysis, the significant positive prognostic factors were well-differentiated NET, a $SUV_{max}$ of 19.3 or more, and a combined treatment with long-acting SMS analogues and radiolabeled SMS analogues. This study thus demonstrated that $SUV_{max}$ correlates with the clinical and pathologic features of NETs and is also an accurate prognostic index.

Taking these factors into consideration, a scoring was devised at the ENETS Center of Excellence, Bad Berka to appropriately select patients for personalized PRRT (influencing decisions on the activity to be administered, number of fractions, time between fractions etc.) This score takes into account various clinical aspects and molecular features, depending on the above-mentioned prerequisites (**Table 2**).[25]

A multidisciplinary team of experienced specialists is required for the appropriate management of patients with NETs. The success of personalized PRRT is determined by appropriate choice of peptide and radionuclide, kidney protection (lysine, arginine, and gelofusine), tumor and organ dosimetry (posttreatment scans), and monitoring of toxicity (follow-up). Above all, appropriate patient selection is the cornerstone of PRRT and presently $^{68}$Ga-SSTR PET/CT using SMS analogues has an unparalleled role.

**Indications/Prerequisites for PRRT**

- Well-differentiated NETs (G1 and G2)
- SSTR expression
- Documented progression of disease with metastasis (in certain cases with high tumor burden without progression might also be considered)
- Inoperability (however, also in neoadjuvant setting, to render an inoperable primary tumor operable)
- For symptomatic improvement in functional NET refractory to octreotide or lanreotide therapy
- Karnofsky index $\geq 60\%$
- Normal renal function and hematological status

## REFERENCES

1. Baum RP, Kulkarni HR, Carreras C. Peptides and receptors in image-guided therapy: theranostics for neuroendocrine neoplasms. Semin Nucl Med 2012; 42:190–207.

2. Keyes JW Jr. SUV: standard uptake or silly useless value? J Nucl Med 1995;36:1836–9.

3. Kaemmerer D, Peter L, Lupp A, et al. Molecular imaging with 68Ga-SSTR PET/CT and correlation to immunohistochemistry of somatostatin receptors in neuroendocrine tumors. Eur J Nucl Med Mol Imaging 2011;8:1659–68.

4. Miederer M, Seidl S, Buck A, et al. Correlation of immunohistopathological expression of somatostatin receptor 2 with standardised uptake values in 68Ga-DOTATOC PET/CT. Eur J Nucl Med Mol Imaging 2009;36:48–52.

5. Müssig K, Oksüz MO, Dudziak K, et al. Association of somatostatin receptor 2 immunohistochemical expression with [111In]-DTPA octreotide scintigraphy and [68Ga]-DOTATOC PET/CT in neuroendocrine tumors. Horm Metab Res 2010;42:599–606.

6. Boy C, Heusner TA, Poeppel TD, et al. 68Ga-DOTATOC PET/CT and somatostatin receptor (sst1-sst5) expression in normal human tissue: correlation of sst2 mRNA and SUV max. Eur J Nucl Med Mol Imaging 2011;38:1224–36.

7. Krenning EP, Kwekkeboom DJ, Bakker WH, et al. Somatostatin receptor scintigraphy with [111In-DTPA-D-Phe1]- and [123I-Tyr3]-octreotide: the Rotterdam experience with more than 1000 patients. Eur J Nucl Med Mol Imaging 1993;20:716–31.

8. Treglia G, Castaldi P, Rindi G, et al. Diagnostic performance of Gallium-68 somatostatin receptor PET and PET/CT in patients with thoracic and gastroenteropancreatic neuroendocrine tumours: a meta-analysis. Endocrine 2012;42:80–7.

9. Hofmann M, Maecke H, Borner R, et al. Biokinetics and imaging with the somatostatin receptor PET radioligand 68Ga-DOTATOC: preliminary data. Eur J Nucl Med Mol Imaging 2001;28:1751–7.

10. Buchmann I, Henze M, Engelbrecht S, et al. Comparison of 68Ga-DOTATOC PET and 111In-DTPAOC (Octreoscan) SPECT in patients with neuroendocrine tumors. Eur J Nucl Med Mol Imaging 2007;34:1617–26.

11. Gabriel M, Decristoforo C, Kendler D, et al. 68Ga-DOTA-Tyr3-octreotide PET in neuroendocrine tumors: comparison with somatostatin receptor scintigraphy and CT. J Nucl Med 2007;48:508–18.

12. Kowalski J, Henze M, Schuhmacher J, et al. Evaluation of positron emission tomography imaging using [68Ga]-DOTA-D Phe(1)-Tyr(3)-octreotide in comparison to [111In]-DTPAOC SPECT. First results in patients with neuroendocrine tumors. Mol Imaging Biol 2003;5:42–8.

13. Srirajaskanthan R, Kayani I, Quigley AM, et al. The role of 68Ga-DOTATATE PET in patients with neuroendocrine tumors and negative or equivocal findings on 111In-DTPA-octreotide scintigraphy. J Nucl Med 2010;51:875–82.

14. Ambrosini V, Campana D, Bodei L, et al. 68Ga-DOTANOC PET/CT clinical impact in patients with neuroendocrine tumors. J Nucl Med 2010;51:669–73.

15. Kayani I, Conry BG, Groves AM, et al. A comparison of 68Ga-DOTATATE and 18F-FDG PET/CT in pulmonary neuroendocrine tumors. J Nucl Med 2009;50:1927–32.

16. Kaemmerer D, Khatib-Chahidi K, Baum RP, et al. Concomitant lung and gastroenteropancreatic neuroendocrine tumors and the value of gallium-68 PET/CT. Cancer Imaging 2011;11:179–83.

17. Prasad V, Ambrosini V, Hommann M, et al. Detection of unknown primary neuroendocrine tumors (CUP-NET) using 68Ga-DOTA-NOC receptor PET/CT. Eur J Nucl Med Mol Imaging 2010;37:67–77.

18. Prasad V, Baum RP. Biodistribution of the Ga-68 labeled somatostatin analogue DOTA-NOC in patients with neuroendocrine tumors: characterization of uptake in normal organs and tumor lesions. Q J Nucl Med Mol Imaging 2010;54:61–7.

19. Severi S, Nanni O, Bodei L, et al. Role of 18FDG PET/CT in patients treated with 177Lu-DOTATATE for advanced differentiated neuroendocrine tumours. Eur J Nucl Med Mol Imaging 2013;40:881–8.

20. Pauwels S, Barone R, Walrand S, et al. Practical dosimetry of peptide receptor radionuclide therapy with (90)Y-labeled somatostatin analogs. J Nucl Med 2005;46(Suppl 1):92S–8S.

21. Kulkarni H, Prasad V, Schuchardt C, et al. Peptide receptor radionuclide therapy (PRRNT) of neuroendocrine tumors: relationship between tumor dose and molecular response as measured by somatostatin receptor PET/CT [abstract]. J Nucl Med 2011;52:301.

22. Ezziddin S, Lohmar J, Yong-Hing CJ, et al. Does the pretherapeutic tumor SUV in 68Ga DOTATOC PET predict the absorbed dose of 177Lu octreotate? Clin Nucl Med 2012;37:e141–7.

23. Singh B, Prasad V, Schuchardt C, et al. Can the standardized uptake values derived from diagnostic 68Ga-DOTATATE PET/CT imaging predict the radiation dose delivered to the metastatic liver NET lesions on 177Lu-DOTATATE peptide receptor radionuclide therapy? J Postgrad Med Educ Res 2013;47:7–13.

24. Campana D, Ambrosini V, Pezzilli R, et al. Standardized uptake values of 68Ga-DOTANOC PET: a promising prognostic tool in neuroendocrine tumors. J Nucl Med 2010;51:353–9.

25. Baum RP, Kulkarni HR. THERANOSTICS: from molecular imaging using Ga-68 labeled tracers and PET/CT to personalized radionuclide therapy - the bad berka experience. Theranostics 2012;2(5):437–47.

# Theranostics with Ga-68 Somatostatin Receptor PET/CT
## Monitoring Response to Peptide Receptor Radionuclide Therapy

Harshad R. Kulkarni, MD*, Richard P. Baum, MD, PhD

## KEYWORDS

• Somatostatin Receptors • Theranostics • Response

## KEY POINTS

- Peptide receptor radionuclide therapy (PRRT) involves selective targeting of neuroendocrine tumors through somatostatin receptors (SSTRs) with the aim to increase radiation dose to the tumors and spare normal tissue.
- The advantage of this internal radiation therapy is the ability to selectively target multiple metastases throughout the body.
- Early and accurate assessment of therapy response helps not only to identify the poor responders but also to personalize the treatment regimens with the aim of achieving maximum treatment benefit.
- Although the evidence regarding utility of [18]F-FDG PET for response assessment after radionuclide therapy is mainly confined to radioimmunotherapy of non-Hodgkin lymphoma, [68]Ga-SSTR PET/computed tomography has a unique theranostic advantage in the assessment of response after PRRT using [177]Lu- or [90]Y-based somatostatin analogues.

## INTRODUCTION

The various modalities available for the monitoring of response to peptide receptor radionuclide therapy (PRRT) in neuroendocrine tumors (NETs) include biochemical, morphologic, and molecular. Chromogranin A has been suggested to be valuable in evaluating the efficacy of a broad range of therapies for NETs, including PRRT.[1,2] Because of its poor sensitivity, however, it may not be reliable and reproducible.[3] Serial measurements of the size of tumor to evaluate the morphologic response to therapy have been standardized, such as by Response Evaluation Criteria in Solid Tumors (RECIST) criteria.[4,5] The major advantage of morphology-based imaging modalities such as computed tomography (CT) or magnetic resonance imaging (MR imaging) is that they are readily available and reproducible. There are several limitations of taking only the morphologic response criteria into account.[6] Firstly, not all types of lesions are measurable and they are also heterogeneous in nature. Secondly, the exact amount of viable tumor may not be fully assessed by using size alone, for example, due to altered anatomy after an intervention. Molecular-targeted therapies may not induce tumor regression in the same way as cytotoxic therapies. The morphologic response criteria lack sensitivity for classifying tumor response when the therapy for which the response is being assessed is cytostatic. Therapy evaluation of

THERANOSTICS Center for Molecular Radiotherapy and Molecular Imaging, ENETS Center of Excellence, Zentralklinik Bad Berka, 99437 Bad Berka, Germany
* Corresponding author.
E-mail address: harshad.kulkarni@zentralklinik.de

PET Clin 9 (2014) 91–97
http://dx.doi.org/10.1016/j.cpet.2013.08.016

slow-growing NETs based on changes in size alone is insufficient. Also, because a high percentage of NETs are nonfunctioning, clinical response parameters may not be adequate. Therefore, a combined imaging approach using molecular response parameter and morphologic information should be more accurate for detection of early treatment response because functional changes at the molecular level may precede the structural changes in disease. Because radionuclide therapy operates at the molecular level, gross morphologic alterations manifest at a later stage. Moreover, unlike many other therapeutic modalities, internal radiation therapy induces damage to tumor cells over a long period. As a consequence, the accumulation of necrotic and fibrotic tissue may cause the size of the lesions to either appear unchanged or even increase, which would be falsely interpreted as stable/progressive with the presently recommended guidelines to use World Health Organization or RECIST criteria to assess response to radionuclide therapy with radiolabeled somatostatin (SMS) analogues in NETs. Because CT or MR imaging may underestimate the therapy response, it has been proposed that stable disease at follow-up be counted as response in patients who were progressing before the commencement of therapy.[7]

## RESPONSE ASSESSMENT USING PET

The recently revised RECIST criteria (RECIST version 1.1) incorporate the information obtained from PET. It was, however, concluded by the RECIST Working Group that there was no sufficient standardization or evidence to abandon anatomic assessment of tumor burden, an exception being with [18]F-FDG, in that it can be used additionally to determine progression.[5] [18]F-FDG uptake is an early and sensitive metabolic imaging parameter to monitor the tumoricidal effect of anticancer drugs. The recommendations on the measurement of [18]F-FDG uptake for tumor response monitoring from a consensus meeting of the European Organization for Research and Treatment of Cancer (EORTC) PET study group were published as the EORTC criteria for metabolic response.[8] A draft framework for PET Response Criteria in Solid Tumors was proposed using the lean body mass–corrected standardized uptake value (SUV) in the hottest tumor focus.[9]

## [68]GA-SOMATOSTATIN RECEPTOR PET/CT

Molecular imaging using somatostatin receptor (SSTR) PET/CT with [68]Ga-labeled SMS analogues and molecular radiotherapy applying PRRT with [90]Y- and/or [177]Lu-labeled peptides is

an excellent example of THERANOSTICS and personalized medicine.[10] Using the identical diagnostic SMS analogue as for therapeutics, SSTR PET/CT using [68]Ga-labeled SMS analogues provides quantitative and reproducible data that can be used for prediction and evaluation of therapy response to PRRT, following the principle of theranostics (Figs. 1–4). However, the potential pitfall of dedifferentiation and loss of SSTR expression by tumors must be taken into account (Fig. 5). Hence despite its limitation, the current evidence-based practice for monitoring of NETs after PRRT takes only the morphologic proof of tumor regression/stabilization rather than a decrease in the tumor uptake per se into account.

One of the earliest studies comparing the molecular and morphologic response criteria was by Gabriel and colleagues,[11] in which PET using [68]Ga-DOTATOC was compared with CT (for response assessment using the RECIST criteria). [68]Ga-DOTATOC PET was performed in 46 patients with advanced NETs who were treated with either [90]Y-DOTA-TOC (n = 24), or [177]Lu-DOTA-octreotate (n = 19), or both compounds (n = 3) before and after 2 to 7 cycles of PRRT. The reference standard used for comparison was CT. A discordance between [68]Ga-DOTATOC PET and CT was observed in 14 patients (30%) with a final outcome of progressive disease in 9 patients and remission in 5 patients. A follow-up [68]Ga-DOTATOC PET detected metastatic spread in 10 patients (21.7%). In 5 of these patients with progressive disease, CT alone would have missed the metastases. On the other hand, CT result was positive and PET result negative in 1 patient with small pulmonary metastases and in 3 patients with progressive liver metastases. Since morphologic response criteria were taken as standard in this study, it was concluded that because change in size was not confirmed in most patients, evaluation of individual lesions on [68]Ga-DOTATOC PET was a poor predictor of progressive disease. Furthermore, evaluation of individual lesions (diameter or SUV) was of no additional value in predicting therapy response, and receptor PET showed no advantage over conventional anatomic imaging for evaluating therapeutic efficacy.

These results were not in conformation with a study by Haug and colleagues.[12] [68]Ga-DOTATATE PET/CT was evaluated for its role in predicting therapeutic response to PRRT at an early stage. It was performed in 33 patients at baseline and 3 months after initiation of the first PRRT cycle. The molecular response was assessed with serial measurements of SUV. The SMS

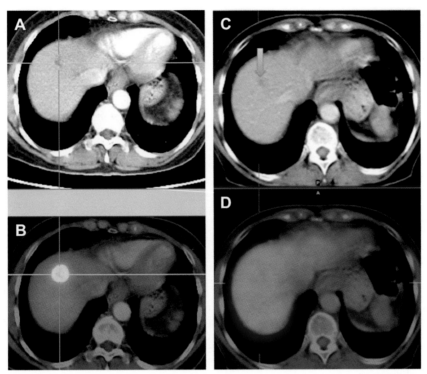

**Fig. 1.** A 65-year-old female patient with pancreatic NET and multiple liver metastases s. p. Whipple operation and Sandostatin therapy, was treated with 5 cycles of PRRT, total administered activity of [90]Y- and [177]Lu-DOTA-TATE (duo-PRRT) 22.6 GBq (611 mCi). As compared to the previous scan before therapy (*A, B*), the post-therapy SSTR PET/CT using [68]Ga-DOTATOC showed a complete remission after the 5th PRRT cycle (*C, D*), according to molecular response criteria. The transverse CT (*A, C*) and fused transverse PET/CT images (*B, D*) are shown here. The response to PRRT is difficult to assess on CT alone, where a hypodense lesion is still noted in segment 8 (*arrow, C*), whereas the fused receptor PET/CT did not demonstrate any significant uptake anymore.

receptor expression was assessed using the maximum SUV ($SUV_{max}$) and tumor-to-spleen SUV ratio (SUV T/S). The percentage change in SUV with respect to the baseline SUV was calculated. The patients were observed for time-to-progression after 1 to 3 cycles of PRRT. Progression was defined on the basis of contrast-enhanced CT and according to RECIST. In addition, the response based on imaging was correlated with clinical symptoms as well as tumor markers chromogranin A and neuron-specific enolase. It was found that decreasing SUV T/S after the first PRRT cycle (in 23 of 31 patients) was associated with a significantly longer progression-free survival (PFS). On the other hand, a reduction in $SUV_{max}$ (in 18 of 33 patients) did not significantly prolong the PFS. In fact, SUV T/S was identified as the only independent predictor for tumor progression during follow-up using multivariate regression analysis, correlating with clinical improvement in the 17 of 33 patients with clinical symptoms before PRRT, whereas $SUV_{max}$ did not. Biochemical response, that is, changes in

biomarkers did not predict SUV scores, clinical improvement, or time to progression. This study showed that a reduction in [68]Ga-DOTATATE uptake in tumors with respect to the spleen (SUV T/S) after the first PRRT cycle predicted time to progression and correlated significantly with an improvement in clinical symptoms.

A pilot study in 138 patients with metastasized, inoperable, well-differentiated NETs (G1 and G2) and evidence of morphologic or clinical progression within the previous year, who underwent 4 cycles of PRRT with an interval of 11 to 16 weeks between successive cycles, demonstrated that assessment of response to PRRT using Ga-68 SSTR PET/CT was useful to predict overall survival (OS) and PFS in patients with NETs. Statistically significant difference was found in the probability of OS after the 4th cycle of PRRNT based on the molecular response status ($P = .021$), as well as in the probability of PFS between patients with PR and those with SD ($P = .034$). However, further studies are required to ascertain this correlation.[13]

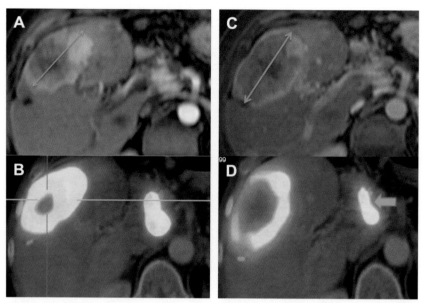

Fig. 2. Transverse T-1 weighted MR imaging before 3rd PRRT cycle (A) in a patient with ileal NET shows a liver metastasis with central necrosis in segment 8. After the 3rd PRRT cycle, there was an increase in size of the lesion (C), however, because of increasing necrosis, which is not possible to quantify with morphologic response parameters alone. The fused [68]Ga-DOTATOC PET/CT images before (B) and after therapy (D) demonstrated a significant decrease in the $SUV_{max}$ in both the liver metastasis (by 55%) and in the lymph node metastasis (arrow, by 42%), indicating partial remission.

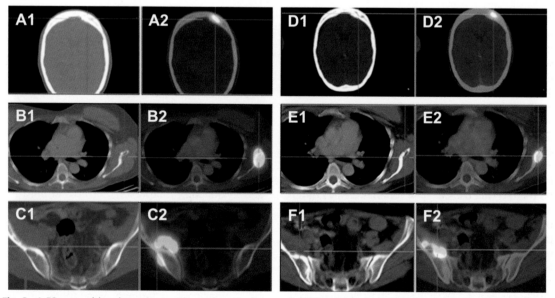

Fig. 3. A 53-year-old male patient with nonfunctioning, well-differentiated, small cell neuroendocrine carcinoma of unknown primary (CUP-NEC) and extensive skeletal metastases was treated with PRRT. The representative [68]Ga-DOTATATE PET/CT transverse images before therapy (A2, B2, C2; A1–C1, corresponding CT) show metastases in the skull (A), left scapula (B), and the right iliac bone (C). After 2 cycles of duo-PRRT with 4.3 GBq [90]Y-DOTATATE and 7 GBq [177]Lu-DOTATATE (with capecitabine) respectively, [68]Ga SSTR PET/CT (D2, E2, F2; D1–F1, corresponding CT) revealed a significant decrease in the $SUV_{max}$ of the 3 target lesions shown here. Clearly, CT alone would have resulted in identification of a stable disease rather than a response.

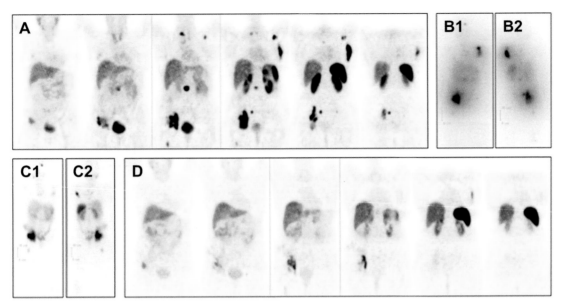

Fig. 4. Molecular response (in the same patient as in Fig. 3) can be well appreciated on coronal receptor PET images before (*A*) and after therapy (*D*). 90Y-DOTATATE whole-body planar Bremsstrahlung scans post-1st PRRT cycle (*B1*, in anterior view and *B2*, in posterior view) as well as 177Lu-DOTATATE whole-body planar scans after the 2nd PRRT (*C1*, in anterior view and *C2*, in posterior view) show high uptake in the above-mentioned target lesions in the skull, left scapula, and right iliac bone.

## ROLE OF ADDITIONAL 18F-FDG PET/CT

18F-fluorodeoxyglucose (FDG) PET has been considered of limited value in evaluating well-differentiated NETs.[14] Garin and colleagues[15] prospectively performed 18F-FDG PET and somatostatin receptor scintigraphy (SRS) in 38 patients with NETs. 18F-FDG PET and SRS results were positive in 15 and 27 patients, respectively. Significantly, early progression was noted in 14 out of 15 18F-FDG PET–positive patients, whereas in only 2 out of the 23 patients who were 18F-FDG–negative. On the other hand, 9 out of 11 SRS-negative patients had early progressive disease as against 7 out of 27 SRS-positive patients. Both 18F-FDG PET and SRS results correlated with PFS and OS even for histologically low-grade tumors, but 18F-FDG PET was in fact the only predictive factor for PFS at multivariate analysis with negative and positive predictive values of 91% and 93%, respectively. Thus, it can predict not only early tumor progression but also changes in tumor biology like dedifferentiation or high-grade transformation during radionuclide therapy. In the study by Gabriel and colleagues,[11] 3 patients with receptor-negative hepatic metastases on a follow-up 68Ga- DOTATOC scan showed enhanced 18F-FDG PET uptake, suggesting of loss of receptor expression and differentiation. Hypermetabolism (18F-FDG PET) and lack of SSTR expression (68Ga-DOTA-TOC) were associated with rapid progression and a short OS, in line with the results of Garin and colleagues.[15] The results were further confirmed by a study investigating the prognostic value of FDG PET in predicting response and PFS after PRRT using 177Lu-DOTATATE (Lu-PRRT) in patients with advanced well-differentiated grade 1/2 NETs.[16] Severi and colleagues concluded that FDG PET evaluation was useful for predicting response because none of the FDG-negative patients had progressed at the first follow-up examination after Lu-PRRT. Grade 2 NET and FDG-positivity (arbitrary SUV cutoff >2.5) were frequently associated with more aggressive disease. Those 32% of grade 2 and FDG-positive patients who did not respond to Lu-PRRT monotherapy might benefit from more intensive therapy protocols, such as the combination of chemotherapy and PRRT.

Thus we postulate that in patients who are eligible for PRRT, SSTR PET as well as 18F-FDG PET may be useful for the early detection of disease progression developing during therapy and also for predicting therapy response. Structural imaging is likely to play an additional pivotal role in the follow-up of NET patients.

## FUTURE PERSPECTIVES

The Bad Berka Molecular Imaging Tool is a new technique under development for automatic segmentation of lesions, which is based on cognition

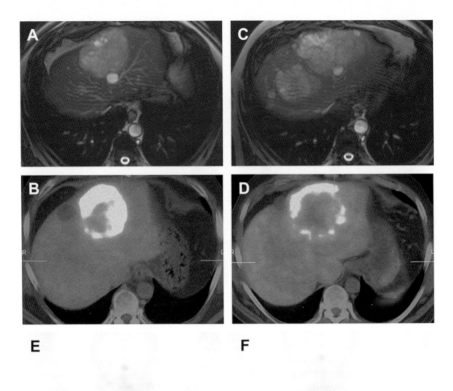

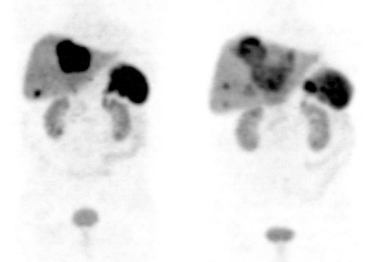

Fig. 5. (*A*) Vanishing somatostatin receptors due to dedifferentiation: A 52-year-old man with well-differentiated (G2, Ki-67 10%), non-functional NET of the pancreatic tail with extensive hepatic metastases was treated with 6 cycles of duo-PRRT, 2nd cycle combining $^{90}$Y- and $^{177}$Lu-DOTATATE (tandem-PRRT), the last cycle in combination with cape-citabine. He was followed-up 2 years after the 6th PRRT, so far with stable disease. However, MR imaging (*A, C*, T2 transverse images; *C*, recent and *A*, previous scan 6 months before) showed progression of disease with increase in size of the target lesion in S4. Several new hepatic and lymph node metastases were seen as well as increased size of the previously noted lesions. In addition, size of the primary tumor in the pancreas had increased along with findings suspicious of splenic and stomach infiltration, and mesenteric vein thrombosis. Thus, it represented a clear picture of progressive disease. Interestingly, abdominal ultrasound (which could be rather subjective) revealed stable disease. But on $^{68}$Ga-SSTR PET/CT (fused transverse images: *D*, recent; *B*, before 6 months), a significant decrease in SUV$_{max}$ by 45% was noted in the target lesion in S4a. These findings, which otherwise could be read as partial remission, must be interpreted with caution and should also be correlated with morphologic examination. The conclusion therefore was dedifferentiation of disease with loss of SSTR expression. A comparison of the $^{68}$Ga-DOTATOC PET/CT MIP images is shown (F represents the most recent and E obtained 6 months before).

network language (CNL, Definiens AG, Munich, Germany).[10] Various molecular (PET/CT) parameters like SUV, molecular tumor volume, molecular tumor diameter (MTD), molecular tumor index (SUV × MTD), and whole-body and organ tumor burden can be quantified by this automated user-independent software.[5] This not only improves the reproducibility but also increases the sensitivity, shortening the time required for reading a PET scan with multiple tumor lesions. The fast and accurate analysis of serial PET/CTs may allow early monitoring of tumor response and assessment of therapeutic efficacy, thereby personalizing patient management.

## REFERENCES

1. Modlin IM, Gustafsson BI, Moss SF, et al. Chromogranin A: biological function and clinical utility in neuro endocrine tumor disease. Ann Surg Oncol 2010;17:2427–43.

2. Lawrence B, Gustafsson BI, Kidd M, et al. The clinical relevance of chromogranin A as a biomarker for gastroenteropancreatic neuroendocrine tumors. Endocrinol Metab Clin North Am 2011;40:111–34.

3. Ardill JE, O'Dorisio TM. Circulating biomarkers in neuroendocrine tumors of the enteropancreatic tract: application to diagnosis, monitoring disease, and as prognostic indicators. Endocrinol Metab Clin North Am 2010;39:777–90.

4. Sohaib SA, Turner B, Hanson JA, et al. CT assessment of tumour response to treatment: comparison of linear, cross-sectional and volumetric measures of tumour size. Br J Radiol 2000;73:1178–84.

5. Eisenhauer EA, Therasse P, Bogaerts J, et al. New response evaluation criteria in solid tumours: revised RECIST guideline (version 1.1). Eur J Cancer 2009; 45:228–47.

6. Baum RP, Prasad V, Hommann M, et al. Receptor PET/CT imaging of neuroendocrine tumors. Recent Results Cancer Res 2008;170:225–42.

7. Sundin A, Rockall A. Therapeutic monitoring of gastroenteropancreatic neuroendocrine tumors: the challenges ahead. Neuroendocrinology 2012;96: 261–71.

8. Young H, Baum R, Cremerius U, et al. Measurement of clinical and subclinical tumour response using [18F]-fluorodeoxyglucose and positron emission tomography: review and 1999 EORTC recommendations. European Organization for Research and Treatment of Cancer (EORTC) PET Study Group. Eur J Cancer 1999;35:1773–82.

9. Wahl RL, Jacene H, Kasamon Y, et al. From RECIST to PERCIST: Evolving Considerations for PET response criteria in solid tumors. J Nucl Med 2009; 50(Suppl 1):122S–50S.

10. Baum RP, Kulkarni HR, Carreras C. Peptides and receptors in image-guided therapy: theranostics for neuroendocrine neoplasms. Semin Nucl Med 2012; 42:190–207.

11. Gabriel M, Oberauer A, Dobrozemsky G, et al. 68Ga-DOTA-Tyr3-octreotide PET for assessing response to somatostatin-receptor-mediated radionuclide therapy. J Nucl Med 2009;50:1427–34.

12. Haug AR, Auernhammer CJ, Wängler B, et al. 68Ga-DOTATATE PET/CT for the early prediction of response to somatostatin receptor-mediated radionuclide therapy in patients with well-differentiated neuroendocrine tumors. J Nucl Med 2010;51:1349–56.

13. Kulkarni HR, Baum RP. Can molecular response after peptide receptor radionuclide therapy predict the overall and progression-free survival? [abstract]. J Nucl Med 2013;54:197.

14. Adams S, Baum R, Rink T, et al. Limited value of fluorine-18 fluorodeoxyglucose positron emission tomography for the imaging of neuroendocrine tumours. Eur J Nucl Med 1998;25:79–83.

15. Garin E, Le Jeune F, Devillers A, et al. Predictive value of 18F-FDG PET and somatostatin receptor scintigraphy in patients with metastatic endocrine tumors. J Nucl Med 2009;50:858–64.

16. Severi S, Nanni O, Bodei L, et al. Role of 18FDG PET/CT in patients treated with 177Lu-DOTATATE for advanced differentiated neuroendocrine tumours. Eur J Nucl Med Mol Imaging 2013;40(6): 881–8.

# Relevance of PET for Pretherapeutic Prediction of Doses in Peptide Receptor Radionuclide Therapy

Matthias Blaickner, PhD, Richard P. Baum, MD

## KEYWORDS

- Peptide receptor radionuclide therapy • Dosimetry • Pretherapeutic treatment planning • PET/CT
- SPECT/CT • Planar imaging • Correlation with clinical response • Radiobiological models

## KEY POINTS

- Dosimetry in radionuclide therapy in general and in peptide receptor radionuclide therapy in particular remains an interesting, and also a disputed, issue.
- Evidence for a dose-response relationship is available, both for normal organs as well as for lesions, but the mean absorbed dose seems to have limitations for describing dose-effect relationships whereas the inclusion of radiobiological models such as the biological effective dose and the equivalent uniform dose yields better correlation with observable response parameters.
- Clinical imaging protocols for $^{86}$Y-DOTATOC are available and their designers have emphasized its better suitability than $^{111}$In-labled surrogates for dose prediction of $^{90}$Y-DOTATOC.
- PET imaging with $^{90}$Y from its internal pair production is a promising field, yielding impressive results for the dosimetry of $^{90}$Y-SIR-Spheres. Applications for PRRT in patients are yet to come.
- PET with $^{68}$Ga-labeled DOTA-peptides is not suitable for dosimetric calculations but could be valuable in the selection of appropriate candidates for PRRT because of correlation of the SUV of lesions with the absorbed dose from therapy.

## DOSIMETRY IN RADIONUCLIDE THERAPY
### State of the Art and Controversies

Dosimetry in radionuclide therapy, its associated benefit and effort, the inherent uncertainties, and the correlation with clinical data, is an ongoing discussion in the scientific community. Unlike the related medical fields of external beam radiotherapy (EBRT) and brachytherapy, in which dose calculations are the key point for treatment planning and the initial assessment of the tumor response,[1–3] dosimetry is still not routinely implemented for radionuclide therapy. Several scientists have raised concerns about the benefit of dosimetric calculations rather than conventional fixed dosing or dosing per kilogram body weight. There exist studies in which the calculated tumor dose failed to predict the tumor response, such as the work of Sharkey and colleagues[4] on radioimmunotherapy for non-Hodgkin lymphoma. Brans and colleagues[5] acknowledged the value of dosimetry in the preclinical phase of radiopharmaceutical development but doubted its clinical use to optimize administered activity for the individual patient. This notion is countered by others, such as Flux and colleagues,[6] who pointed out that the large variation of the tumor delivered dose in individual patients as reported in numerous studies[7,8]

Health & Environment Department, Biomedical Systems, AIT Austrian Institute of Technology, Donau-City-Strasse 1/2, Vienna A-1220, Austria
E-mail address: matthias.blaickner@ait.ac.at

PET Clin 9 (2014) 99–112
http://dx.doi.org/10.1016/j.cpet.2013.08.014
1556-8598/14/$ – see front matter © 2014 Elsevier Inc. All rights reserved.

highlights an urgent need for tailoring treatment design to the individual case with the aim of maximizing tumor cell kill and minimizing nontarget organ toxicity. This approach would allow radionuclide therapy to reveal its full potential as an important cancer treatment modality.[6]

The available evidence in the literature shows that 2 major findings are evolving. First, more and more studies are showing the existence of dose-effect relationships in clinical practice, such as bone-marrow toxicity for non-Hodgkin lymphoma radioimmunotherapy,[9] metaiodobenzylguanidine treatment of neuroblastoma,[10] and treatment efficacy in radioiodine ablation in differentiated thyroid cancer.[11] Likewise Shen and colleagues[12] concluded in an earlier study that the marrow dose is a better predictor for myelotoxicity than millicuries per square meter or lean total body dose, an insight also confirmed by the work of Siegel and colleagues.[13] These studies showed that even a basic dosimetric methodology such as the absorbed dose provides clinically important data.

However, the second major insight with regard to dosimetry in radionuclide therapy is the significantly improved dose-effect relationship if three-dimensional (3D) voxel-based dosimetry is combined with radiobiological models (**Box 1**). This improved relationship can be best appreciated from the numerous investigations involving thyroid cancer treatment with [131]I, for which lesion-based dosimetry applying [124]I PET imaging is considered the state-of-the-art approach.[14] The research group at the Division of Nuclear Medicine at the Johns Hopkins University has published several research articles that show the value of the analysis of the 3D tumor dose distribution for the response prediction. In an early work,[15] no dose-response relationship for tumors was found after applying patient-specific, voxel-based 3D dosimetry. However, by incorporating the spatial absorbed dose distribution (ie, the dose-volume histograms [DVHs]) into the equivalent uniform dose (EUD) model the tumor response's dependence on the dose nonuniformity was proved.[16] The benefit of this model compared with the mean absorbed tumor dose was confirmed in subsequent studies[17] and also in the case of [131]I-tositumomab radioimmunotherapy,[18] the treatment of high-risk osteosarcoma with [153]Sm-ethylenediamine tetramethylene phosphonic acid,[19] and treatment planning of hepatocellular carcinoma with [90]Y-microspheres,[20] proving that the benefit of 3D tumor dosimetry is not confined to thyroid cancer and/or specifically radionuclide [131]I.

Individual organ dosimetry is also essential for critical organs in order to prevent radiotoxicities. In particular, renal toxicity has been shown to be the major dose-limiting factor in radionuclide therapy.[21] Baechler and colleagues[22] suggested the extension of the BED schema in order to facilitate the investigation of dose-toxicity correlations. In *MIRD Pamphlet No. 20*[23] it is stated that the usage of a multiregional kidney dosimetry model together with the BED makes the radiation dose-response data from radionuclide therapy consistent with the external beam experience for predicting kidney toxicity.

### Dosimetry in Peptide Receptor Radionuclide Therapy

Peptide receptor radionuclide therapy (PRRT) is one of the subcategories of radionuclide therapy and has proved to be an efficient treatment of neuroendocrine tumors (NET) with good clinical and objective response rates. In their recent review, Kam and colleagues[24] pointed out the encouraging results in terms of tumor regression, overall survival, and the improvement in the patient's quality of life. As with the other forms of radionuclide therapy, the correlation between tumor response and absorbed radiation dose is evident. Pauwels and Barone[25] contributed an important study[26] in which they showed that an accurate dosimetry estimation of the kidney, taking into account the BED and individual renal volume, enables prediction of risk of renal function impairment. This finding was taken a step further recently by incorporating radiobiological dosimetry models (discussed earlier). The approach was found to be the best choice for dosimetry of kidneys in PRRT.[27] Another clinical study showed that individual dosimetry should be

---

**Box 1**
**Dosimetric quantities (for the detailed mathematical definitions, see Table 3 of Ref.[21])**

Mean absorbed dose: the energy deposited by ionizing radiation per unit mass of an anatomic structure (eg, organ, tumor). This quantity is averaged for the mass and the irradiation time.

Biologic effective dose (BED): accounts for differences in dose rate (ie, the effective half-life of the radiopharmaceutical) and incorporates the repair half-time for sublethal tissue damage, the average doubling time for tumor clonogenic cells, as well as the assumed intrinsic radiosensitivity.

Equivalent uniform (biological effective) dose (EUD): models the impact of the spatial dose distribution on the response. The BED of each voxel is used to generate an EUD value for a specified volume (eg, organ, tumor).

performed for each individual PRRT cycle because of the large interpatient variability.[28] With regard to the tumor response's dependence on the dose nonuniformity evidence for PRRT is available,[25] albeit limited.

## Dosimetric Imaging in PRRT

The treatment of differentiated thyroid cancer with [131]I shows the usefulness of PET/computed tomography (CT) systems for pretherapeutic dose assessment, using [124]I and [131]I as a beta couple.[14] The beta plus nuclide [124]I is used for PET imaging, which yields the temporal and spatial activity distribution. With regard to dose calculations of the therapeutic beta minus nuclide [131]I, the same biokinetics can be assumed because of identical chemical properties. The comparable physical half-lives (4.5 days for [124]I and 8 days for [131]I) in combination with an effective half-life of 10 to 15 hours[29] prevent a premature cutoff of the time-activity curves. However, such an advantageous combination of factors is not available for PET image–based dosimetry in PRRT. In PRRT, the tracers most frequently applied in therapy are [90]Y-DOTATOC and [90]Y-DOTATATE as well as [177]Lu-DOTATOC and [177]Lu-DOTATATE.[21,24] DOTATOC is the abbreviated form of [DOTA0,Tyr3]-octreotide, where DOTA stands for the bifunctional chelating molecule 1,4,7,10-tetraazacyclo-dodecane-1,4,7,10-tetraacetic acid, and Tyr3-octreotide is the modified octreotide. DOTATATE is the abbreviated form of [DOTA0,Tyr3,Thr8]-octreotide or [DOTA0,Tyr3]-octreotate, and DOTA stands for the bifunctional metalchelating molecule. [111]In was also tested as a therapeutic nuclide for both aforementioned peptides[30,31] but had little success, presumably because of the small range

of the auger electrons, which fail to damage the DNA sufficiently. For dosimetry a collection of serial, planar scintigraphies or single-photon emission computed tomography (SPECT) images are frequently applied, using the [111]In-labeled analogue of the peptide used in therapy,[21,25] [90]Y-bremsstrahlung SPECT/CT images,[32] or SPECT/CT scans acquired during a treatment cycle with [177]Lu-DOTATOC or [177]Lu-DOTATATE.[24,28]

For pretherapeutic prediction of doses in PRRT, PET is not the first choice. Nevertheless, some imaging protocols yield useful information and have potential for further development. **Table 1** provides a summary of the radionuclides whose use is discussed later.

## PET IMAGING TECHNIQUES AND PRACTICES
### [86]Y

### PET imaging of [86]Y

The positron emission branching of [86]Y amounts to 31.9% with the remaining part decaying by electron capture.[33] However, for PET imaging there is also the emission of 75% prompt γ-rays per decay with an energy that is included in the PET energy window as well as 231% high-energy prompt γ-rays with an energy ranging from 650 to 3900 keV.[34] High-energy prompt γ-rays can be scattered down to the PET energy window and cause spurious coincidences just as 2 prompt γ-ray lines from the same decay give way to projection lines that do not include the decay location because the photons were emitted at an angle other than 180°. These false coincidences cause an activity overestimation, which is why in [86]Y-PET imaging special corrections have to be applied that differ from those used for [124]I or [76]Br.[34-36] The suggested methods involve the subtraction of a background

---

**Table 1**
**PET nuclides for dose assessment in PRRT**

| Nuclide | [86]Y | [90]Y | [68]Ga | [44]Sc |
|---|---|---|---|---|
| Half-life | 14.7 h | 64.1 h | 68 min | 3.9 h |
| $E_{max}$ β (MeV) | 0.25–3.14 | 2.28 | 2.92 | 1.48 |
| $E_{mean}$ β (MeV) | 0.11–1.44 | 0.93 | 0.84 | 0.63 |
| β+ branch (%) | 31.9 | 0.003 | 89.1 | 94.3 |
| E γ (MeV) (%) | 0.30–3.33 (348) | 2.19 (0.0001) | 0.22–2.82 (3.4) | 1.16 (99.9) |
| Radiopeptides used for dosimetry | DOTATOC | — | DOTATOC, DOTANOC, DOTATATE | DOTATOC |
| Use | Prediction for [90]Y dosimetry | Direct [90]Y dosimetry | Selection of patients because of correlation with [177]Lu dose | Prediction for [90]Y dosimetry? |

Abbreviation: E, Energy.

that is modeled uniformly,[37,38] linearly,[38,39] or by means of a second-order series expansion.[40] Furthermore, a subtraction based on a convolution with a scatter kernel was suggested by Beattie and colleagues[41] and further developed by Walrand and colleagues,[35] who achieved promising results using a patient-dependent, empirical kernel approach validated by comparison with collected urine activity, a method that has only been tested for two-dimensional (2D) acquisitions. In 3D the spurious coincidences are supposed to increase significantly. Moreover, a narrower energy window reduces the random coincidence rates of high-energy γ-rays and thus can help improve the image quality. However, this may increase the inaccuracy of the dead time corrections as shown by Kull and colleagues.[40]

### Dosimetry based on [86]Y-petides

[111]In-DOTATOC, images have been used in clinical practice[42] in order to calculate the dosimetry of [90]Y-DOTATOC therapies. Analogous to the aforementioned beta-couple [124]I and [131]I for thyroid cancer, [86]Y-DOTATOC can be applied to predict the dosimetry of a [90]Y-based PRRT. The advantage is

the improved spatial resolution and absolute quantification of PET imaging, which has to be counted against the high level of noise from the prompt γ emissions, the challenges and costs in obtaining [86]Y and (most severe) the short physical half-life of 14.7 hours compared with 64.1 hours for [90]Y, which results in a time window for data collection of about 24 to 40 hours[43] and limits the pharmacokinetic data of late time points and consequently has an impact on the accuracy of the dose calculations. Nevertheless multiple studies show the superior image quality and quantification process of [86]Y-labeled DOTA peptides compared with [111]In-labeled tracers (Fig. 1).[25,44–46]

**Box 2** provides a short bulleted list on [86]Y-PET and **Table 2** gives an overview of the imaging protocols used. The patients in these studies all had a metastatic– NET and ranged from 41 to 75 years of age. In all cases the PET tracer was [86]Y-DOTATOC, measured in 2D mode.

### Summaries drawn from [86]Y-based dosimetry
Barone and colleagues[26] concluded that [86]Y-DOTATOC in combination with the BED model of the kidney can be used successfully for

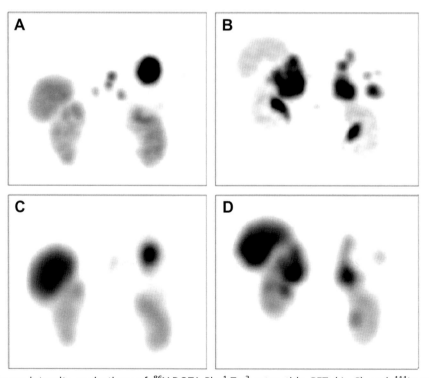

**Fig. 1.** Maximum intensity projections of [86]Y-DOTA-Phe[1]-Tyr[3]-octreotide PET (*A, B*) and [111]In-pentetreotide SPECT (*C, D*) 24 hours after injection in posterior views: patient no. 1 (*A, C*) and patient no. 2 (*B, D*). [86]YDOTA-Phe[1]-Tyr[3]-octreotide reveals more metastases than [111]In-pentetreotide. Kidney and spleen uptake appears higher in the [111]In-pentetreotide scans than in the [86]Y-DOTA-Phe[1]-Tyr[3]-octreotide PET scans. (*From* Helisch A, Förster GJ, Reber H, et al. Pre-therapeutic dosimetry and biodistribution of 86Y-DOTA-Phe1-Tyr3-octreotide versus 111In-pentetreotide in patients with advanced neuroendocrine tumours. Eur J Nucl Med Mol Imaging 2004;31(10):1389; with permission.)

Inclusion criteria:

- Patient 18 years of age or older
- Histologically confirmed NET
- Somatostatin receptor positive

Data acquisition:

- Correction of spurious coincidences
- 2D acquisition mode
- Blood and urine samples advantageous for dosimetry
- Kidney protection: coinfusion of amino acid over 4 hours, starting 30 minutes before injection
- Patients should drink 2 to 3 L a day

accurate dosimetry of 90Y-DOTATOC, predicting the risk of renal impairment. Förster and colleagues[46] recommend the usage of 86Y-DOTATOC rather than 111In-DTPA-octreotide for pretherapeutic dosimetry of 90Y-DOTATOC, and Helisch and colleagues[45] described it as the gold standard. However, critical investigators point out the difficulties caused by the short half-life, high cost, and low availability[21] and argue that 86Y-based surrogate imaging can provide important scientific information on doses to tumors and organs but is not suitable for individual therapy planning (ie, the optimization of the injected activity).[34]

## 90Y

### PET imaging of 90Y
90Y-Imaging is usually associated with the bremsstrahlung radiographs originating from its beta

Table 2
Parameters of 86Y-DOTATOC imaging protocols

| Study | Barone et al,[26] 2005 | Förster et al,[46] 2001 | Helisch et al,[45] 2004 | Jamar et al,[47] 2003 |
|---|---|---|---|---|
| Injected activity (MBq) | 286 ± 119 | 77–186; mean, 137 | 254–394; mean, 310 | 122–385 |
| Coinfusion | Amino acid | None | Amino acid | Amino acid |
| Scans | 3.5, 24, and 48 h after injection | 45 min dynamic scan starting at time of injection; scans of thorax and abdomen 1, 2, 4, 6, 10, 20, 30, and 48 h after injection | 1, 4, 24, 30, and 48 h after injection | 3.5, 24, and 48 h after injection |
| Bed positions | 10 at 3.5 h; 3–6 at 24 and 48 h | 3–4 | 2–3 | 10 at 3.5 h; 3–6 at 24 and 48 h |
| Reconstruction | OSEM | FBP with Hanning filter | OSEM | OSEM |
| Biokinetic fit | Linear between 4 and 24 h, extrapolated to time 0, monoexponential function between 24 and 48 h used for washout | Triexponential curves | Triexponential curves | Linear between 4 and 24 h, extrapolated to time 0, monoexponential function between 24 and 48 h used for washout |
| Dosimetry | MIRDOSE: ROIs on PET, individual kidney volume from CT, BED for kidney | MIRDOSE: ROIs on PET (including tumor), activity concentration in blood and urine | MIRDOSE: ROIs on PET (including tumor), activity concentration in blood and urine | MIRDOSE: ROIs on PET (including tumor), activity concentration in blood and urine |

Abbreviations: FBP, filtered back projection; MIRDOSE, Medical Internal Radiation Dose; OSEM, ordered subset expectation maximization; ROI, region of interest.
Data from Refs.[26,45–47]

minus spectrum, which has a high end point energy (2.2 MeV) and can therefore be detected by gamma cameras and used for SPECT.[32,48–50] However the existence of a $0^+$ - $0^+$ transition results in an internal pair production of electron and positron with a small probability of $34 \pm 4 \times 10^{-6}$.[51] In 2004, Nickels and colleagues[52] were the first to produce PET images of $^{90}$Y biodistribution and soon were followed by others. Werner and colleagues[53] used a PET system with lutetium oxyorthosilicate (LSO) crystals to assess $^{90}$Y distribution after selective internal radiotherapy (SIRT) of liver metastases. Gates and colleagues[54] also used a conventional PET/CT system for the localization of $^{90}$Y glass microspheres.

Comparisons between $^{90}$Y-PET and SPECT have reached different conclusions. Rault and colleagues[55] achieved a PET spatial resolution of 6.4 mm compared with 15.3 mm for SPECT, but emphasized that the count rate was 6.25 times higher for SPECT, which in turn requires specific correction for the bremsstrahlung. Fabbri and colleagues[56] came to the conclusion that $^{90}$Y-SPECT/CT is the method of choice for clinical applications such as systemic infusion and that PET with $^{90}$Y is not suitable for that despite its better spatial resolution. However, the introduction of time of flight (TOF) to $^{90}$Y-PET adds another facet to the discussion. Lhommel and colleagues[57] showed that $^{90}$Y-TOF PET supersedes $^{90}$Y-bremsstrahlung SPECT and correlates well with $^{18}$F-fluorodeoxyglucose (FDG)-PET and CT scans (**Fig. 2**). In their acquisition of a patient receiving 1.3 GBq of SIR-Spheres they used a 2.5-mm copper ring to shield the bremsstrahlung x-rays. Furthermore, Elschot and colleagues[58] stated that TOF PET not only provides a superior image quality to bremsstrahlung SPECT but also results in more accurate dose estimates.

Van Elmbt and colleagues[59] compared an lutetium yttrium orthosilicate (LYSO). TOF PET and 2 gadolinium oxyorthosilicate (GSO) and bismuth germinate (BGO) non-TOF PET scanners by means of a phantom simulating liver SIRT. The

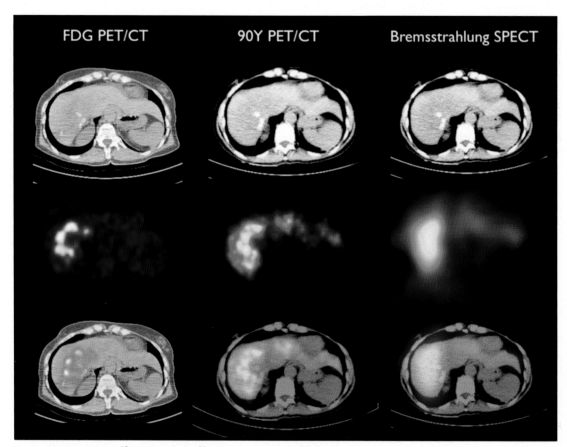

**Fig. 2.** Comparison of $^{18}$F-FDG-PET/CT, $^{90}$Y TOF PET/CT, and $^{90}$Y-SPECT/CT of a 61-year-old woman with colorectal liver metastasis. Data were reconstructed using OSEM (4 iterations, 6 subsets). (*From* Lhommel R, Goffette P, Van den Eynde M, et al. Yttrium-90 TOF PET scan demonstrates high-resolution biodistribution after liver SIRT. Eur J Nucl Med Mol Imaging 2009;36(10):1696; with permission.)

LYSO TOF PET yielded the best results, whereas conventional LYSO and GSO showed a decrease in contrast. The quality of BGO imaging was insufficient for dosimetry calculation.

## Dosimetry based on $^{90}$Y-PET

Considering the relative young age of $^{90}$Y-PET imaging, available data on dosimetric imaging studies are sparse. Lhommel and colleagues[60] imaged $^{90}$Y-labeled SIR-Spheres using 3D LYSO TOF PET without a copper ring and showed the sensitivity to be linear up to 2.5 GBq. Furthermore, dosimetry calculations using $^{90}$Y voxel S values agreed with concurrent calculations performed with Organ Level Internal Dose Assessment (OLINDA) (**Fig. 3**).[61] Contrary to the findings of Van Elmbt and colleagues[59] mentioned earlier, D'Arienzo and colleagues[62] considered a PET/CT scanner with BGO crystals to be a reliable system for the dose assessment of liver SIRT treatment and showed a correlation between absorbed dose and tumor response.

PET imaging has not yet been used for patients undergoing $^{90}$Y-PRRT, but pioneering work was performed by Walrand and colleagues[63] in measuring a fillable kidney phantom based on the MIRD kidney model[64] as well as vertebrae with attenuation similar to that of bone and spheres simulating tumors. The $^{90}$Y activity amounted to 4.4 GBq, which is a typical uptake for the first $^{90}$Y-DOTATOC cycle. Eight successive 45-minute scans were acquired on a TOF LYSO as well as a

BGO system and the dosimetry was assessed in 4 steps, including the determination of the recovery coefficient by means of a point-spread function. The results showed that both PET systems were able to accurately determine the tumor dose and that BGO showed a smaller deviation than TOF LYSO with regard to renal dosimetry, which was ascribed to the natural radioactivity in the crystal. However, another relevant finding of this study was that neither system could provide an accurate red marrow dosimetry.

## $^{68}$Ga

### Correlations of $^{68}$Ga uptake with absorbed $^{177}$Lu dose

The positron branching ratio of $^{68}$Ga is ~89% with a total probability for γ-emission of only ~ 3.4%.[33] $^{68}$Ga-labeled DOTA-peptides have become an indispensable component in the diagnosis and management of NETs. Detailed discussions on imaging protocols and best practice are given in Refs.[65–69] However, because of the short half-life of $^{68}$Ga (68 minutes) compared with the effective half-life of the peptides used for therapy, it is not suitable to measure the washout trend of the time-activity curves.[43] Nevertheless a high standardized uptake value (SUV) of a $^{68}$Ga tracer in a specific lesion is associated with a high uptake of the therapeutic $^{90}$Y or $^{177}$Lu counterpart, which consequently is expected to result in a high radiation dose. A few research teams[70–72] have examined this correlation by comparing the SUVs of

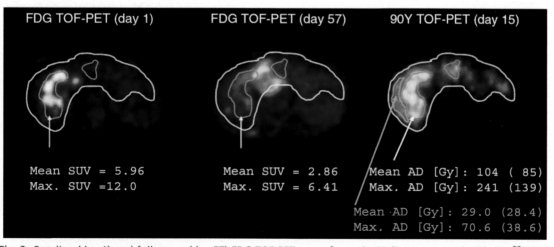

**Fig. 3.** Baseline (day 1) and follow-up (day 57) FDG TOF PET scan of a patient's liver compared with the $^{90}$Y TOF PET raw activity distribution measured after $^{90}$Y-labeled SIR-Spheres therapy (day 15). Tumor response was noted in the region of high absorbed dose (AD; 104 Gy), whereas a tumor progression occurred in the region not targeted by the $^{90}$Y-labeled SIR-Spheres. ADs were computed using the $^{90}$Y 4-mm voxel S values with spatial resolution deconvolution (SRD) and in parentheses without SRD or recovery coefficients. (SUV = standardized uptake value). (*From* Lhommel R, van Elmbt L, Goffette P, et al. Feasibility of 90Y TOF PET-based dosimetry in liver metastasis therapy using SIR-Spheres. Eur J Nucl Med Mol Imaging 2010;37(9):1660; with permission.)

$^{68}$Ga-labeled DOTA-peptides with the absorbed doses assessed for the therapeutic cycles using $^{177}$Lu. **Table 3** gives an overview of the different imaging protocols as well as dosimetric and statistical methodologies. All studies examined patients with documented, metastatic NET, whereas Singh and colleagues[71] only considered liver metastasis in their evaluation (**Fig. 4**). With regard to the PET acquisition, the 3D mode was used.

**Table 4** compares the average for all lesions with regard to the $SUV_{max}$, $SUV_{mean}$, and the absorbed dose per administered activity as well as the correlation coefficients. The SUVs and absorbed doses display good agreement, especially between Ezziddin and colleagues[70] and Singh and colleagues.[71] There is a strong correlation between SUVs and absorbed dose in the studies of Ezziddin and colleagues and Scheler and colleagues,[72] whereas Singh and colleagues[71] observed almost no correlation. However, Ezziddin and colleagues achieved a strong correlation using different peptides for PET imaging and $^{177}$Lu therapy (DOTATOC and DOTATATE), whereas Singh and colleagues,[71] for most

---

**Table 3**
**Imaging parameters, dosimetry, and statistical methods used in studies examining the correlation between SUV of $^{68}$Ga and absorbed dose from $^{177}$Lu**

| Study | Ezziddin et al,[70] 2011 | Singh et al,[71] 2013 | Scheler et al,[72] 2012 |
|---|---|---|---|
| No. patients | 21 (10 male, 11 female) | 12 (8 male, 4 female) | 6 (4 male, 2 female) |
| No. lesions | 61 | 27 | 15 |
| Age (y) | Mean, 69; range: 50–85 | Mean, 60; range: 23–78 | No information available |
| **PET** | | | |
| Peptide | DOTATOC | DOTATATE (10) DOTATOC (1) DOTANOC (1) | DOTATATE |
| Injected activity (MBq) | 117.3 ± 33.9 | 130 ± 18.5 | 150–250 |
| Acquisition time after injection (min) | 75 ± 15.4 | 72.9 ± 12.0 | 60 |
| Scan time per bed position (min) | 4 | 1–2 | No information available |
| **CT** | | | |
| Voltage (kV) | 130 | 130 | No information available |
| Electric charge (mAs) | 60 | 115 | No information available |
| Slice thickness (mm) | 5 | 5 | No information available |
| **$^{177}$Lu imaging** | | | |
| Device | Dual-head gamma camera | Dual-head gamma camera | SPECT/CT |
| Peptide | DOTATATE | DOTATATE | DOTATATE |
| Injected activity (GBq) | 7.47 ± 1.39 | 6.71 ± 0.66 | 3.0–7.7 |
| Acquisition times after injection (h) | 24, 48, 192 | 3, 20, 44, 68 | 15, 40, 64 |
| **Dosimetry** | | | |
| Biokinetic fit | Monoexponential | Monoexponential and biexponential | Monoexponential |
| Dose model for lesions | Sphere module (OLINDA/EXM) | Sphere module (OLINDA/EXM) | Voxel basis (Phillips STRATOS) |
| Statistical test for correlation | Spearman | Spearman | No information available |

*Abbreviation:* OLINDA/EXM, Organ Level Internal Dose Assessment with Exponential Modeling.
   *Data from* Refs.[70–72]

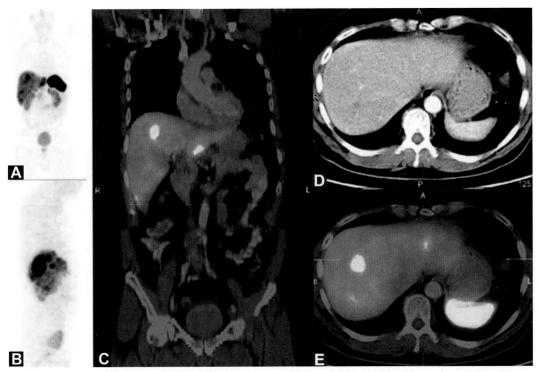

**Fig. 4.** $^{68}$Ga-DOTATATE PET/CT maximum intensity projection (*A, B*), coronal fused (*C*), axial CT (*D*), and corresponding axial fused (*E*) images showing multiple areas of focal tracer uptake in the liver. (*Courtesy of* Prof. Richard P. Baum, Bad Berka, Germany.)

patients, used the same peptide and achieved no significant correlation.

*Future perspectives*
Further studies are required with larger numbers of patients in order to examine this phenomenon. The studies cited earlier have some limitations in their methodology that should be overcome in future work. Two of 3 applied dosimetry from planar, 2D imaging data. However, 3D dosimetry should be based on 3D tomographic images, as done by Scheler and colleagues,[72] who also performed voxel-based dosimetry. As discussed earlier, the important value of fine-resolution, image-based dosimetry is the generation of DVHs and their

subsequent incorporation into radiobiological models, which makes it possible to examine correlations between the SUVs and dosimetric quantities such as the BED and the EUD that have proved to have a higher clinical significance than the absorbed dose.[16,17] A significant correlation could be very valuable in the selection of appropriate candidates for PRRT.

In addition, the comparison of the analysis of a diagnostic PET/CT and a posttherapy SPECT/CT of the same patient allows study of the dependence of the tracer's tumor uptake behavior on the total amount of activity administered, because in a therapeutic application this quantity is an order of magnitude higher, whereas at the same time the

**Table 4**
**Comparison of PET uptake, lesion dose, and its correlation**

| Study | Ezziddin et al,[70] 2011 | Singh et al,[71] 2013 | Scheler et al,[72] 2012 |
|---|---|---|---|
| SUV$_{max}$ | 24.0 ± 14.6 | 21.4 ± 13.1 | 5–189 |
| SUV$_{mean}$ | 13.7 ± 7.3 | 12.6 ± 7.4 | 4–155 |
| D/A$_0$ (Gy/GBq) | 9.0 ± 7.7 | 9.7 ± 7.3 | 0.45–12.4 |
| r (SUV$_{max}$ − D/A$_0$) | 0.71 | 0.039 | 0.79 |
| r (SUV$_{mean}$ − D/A$_0$) | 0.72 | 0.007 | 0.76 |

*Abbreviations:* r, correlation coefficient; D/A$_0$, lesion dose per unit administered activity.
*Data from* Refs.[70–72]

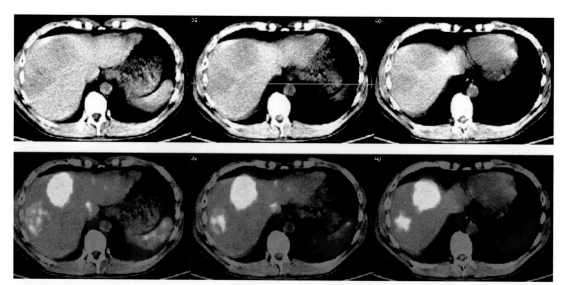

**Fig. 5.** PET/CT imaging of somatostatin receptor–positive liver metastases 18 hours after administration of 37 MBq of $^{44}$Sc-DOTATOC (first in human use). (*From* Rösch F, Baum RP. Generator-based PET radiopharmaceuticals for molecular imaging of tumors: on the way to THERANOSTICS. Dalton Trans 2011;40(23):6110; with permission.)

receptor density of tumor cells presumably stays the same. Animal studies have shown the influence of a diagnostic versus therapeutic quantity on tumor kinetics.[73]

### $^{44}$Sc: a New Outlook?

$^{44}$Sc is discussed briefly here, because it is a nuclide that just recently been introduced in PET imaging. It has a positron branching ratio of 94%, a $\gamma$-line of 1157 keV, and 99.9% intensity.[33] With a half-life of 3.92 hours it is a potential candidate for the cases of PET imaging that require a longer observation time than the narrow time window of $^{68}$Ga, such as the pre-therapeutic imaging for prediction of doses in PRRT. Koumarianou and colleagues[74] managed to synthesize $^{44}$Sc-DOTA-BN$^{2-14}$NH$_2$ as well as $^{68}$Ga-DOTA-BN$^{2-14}$NH$_2$ and studied their biodistribution in normal rats. In spite of the different receptor affinity, the molecules displayed comparable biokinetics and an equal tumor uptake.

The first use in humans was by Rösch and Baum[75] who synthesized $^{44}$Sc-DOTATOC and showed the somatostatin localization of G-protein–coupled transmembrane tumor receptors in patient studies (**Fig. 5**), having a high quality of PET/CT images even 18 hours after injection. As a chemically analogous tracer to $^{90}$Y-DOTATOC and $^{177}$Lu-DOTATOC, $^{44}$Sc-DOTATOC could be used to predict the dosimetry for PRRT.

### SUMMARY

Dosimetry in radionuclide therapy in general, and in PRRT in particular, remains an interesting and also disputed issue. Evidence for a dose-response relationship is available, both for normal organs as well as for lesions, but the quantity of the mean absorbed dose seems to have limitations in describing dose-effect relationships. The inclusion of radiobiological models such as the BED and the EUD yields better correlation with observable response parameters and therefore will, sooner or later, most likely be introduced into clinical dose assessment protocols. However, for these models, the standard MIRD dosimetry applying OLINDA/EXM (or its former version MIRDOSE) is not applicable but requires an image-based, 3D, voxel-by-voxel dosimetry approach whose clinical implementation and application are more complex and time consuming.

Although in principle PET is better for quantitative imaging and has a better spatial resolution than SPECT, in PRRT the latter is currently used for this advanced form of dosimetry. This dosimetry is achieved by scans during a $^{177}$Lu-DOTA-peptide therapy, applying bremsstrahlung imaging for a $^{90}$Y tracer or using $^{111}$In as its surrogate. This does not mean that PET should be written off with regard to dose assessment in PRRT in a broader sense.

Clinical imaging protocols for $^{86}$Y-DOTATOC are available and their designers have emphasized its better suitability than $^{111}$In-labled surrogates for dose prediction of $^{90}$Y-DOTATOC because of the identical chemical properties. This recommendation comes at the price of a short half-life and the effort to correct for the high amount of spurious coincidences.

PET imaging with $^{90}$Y from its internal pair production is a promising field, yielding impressive results for the dosimetry of $^{90}$Y-SIR-Spheres. Applications for PRRT in patients are yet to come, but they will enable three-dimensional acquisition to accompany therapy (as with $^{177}$Lu and SPECT) and will also bring advantages with regard to the protection of clinical staff from radiation, because no additional imaging has to be performed and $^{90}$Y causes a low dose rate outside the patient. The failure in the prediction of the red marrow dose can be compensated by alternative approaches, such as measuring the decrease of platelet counts.[76]

PET with $^{68}$Ga-labeled DOTA-peptides, the gold standard for diagnosis in NET, is not suitable for dosimetric calculations but could be valuable in the selection of appropriate candidates for PRRT because of correlation of the SUV of lesions measured in PET with the absorbed dose from therapy. This phenomenon was observed by 2 studies and contradicted by 1, calling for the analysis of larger series and the inclusion of radiobiological dose quantities in the statistical check for correlations.

$^{44}$Sc can be coupled to DOTA-peptides and may eventually be used for pretherapeutic dose assessment in PRRT. However, this technology is still in its infancy.

## REFERENCES

1. Georg P, Pötter R, Georg D, et al. Dose effect relationship for late side effects of the rectum and urinary bladder in magnetic resonance image-guided adaptive cervix cancer brachytherapy. Int J Radiat Oncol Biol Phys 2012;82(2):653–7.

2. Dunavoelgyi R, Dieckmann K, Gleiss A, et al. Local tumor control, visual acuity, and survival after hypofractionated stereotactic photon radiotherapy of choroidal melanoma in 212 patients treated between 1997 and 2007. Int J Radiat Oncol Biol Phys 2011; 81(1):199–205.

3. Wulf J, Baier K, Mueller G, et al. Dose-response in stereotactic irradiation of lung tumors. Radiother Oncol 2005;77(1):83–7.

4. Sharkey RM, Brenner A, Burton J, et al. Radioimmunotherapy of Non-Hodgkin's lymphoma with 90Y-DOTA humanized anti-CD22 IgG (90Y-epratuzumab): do tumor targeting and dosimetry predict therapeutic response? J Nucl Med 2003;44(12):2000–18.

5. Brans B, Bodei L, Giammarile F, et al. Clinical radionuclide therapy dosimetry: the quest for the 'Holy Gray'. Eur J Nucl Med Mol Imaging 2007; 34(5):772–86.

6. Flux G, Bardies M, Chiesa C, et al. Clinical radionuclide therapy dosimetry: the quest for the 'Holy Gray'. Eur J Nucl Med Mol Imaging 2007;34(10): 1699–700.

7. Matthay KK, Panina C, Huberty J, et al. Correlation of tumor and whole-body dosimetry with tumor response and toxicity in refractory neuroblastoma treated with (131)I-MIBG. J Nucl Med 2001; 42(11):1713–21.

8. Sgouros G, Kolbert KS, Sheikh A, et al. Patient-specific dosimetry for 131I thyroid cancer therapy using 124I PET and 3-dimensional-internal dosimetry (3D-ID) software. J Nucl Med 2004;45(8): 1366–72.

9. Ferrer L, Kraeber-Bodéré F, Bodet-Milin C, et al. Three methods assessing red marrow dosimetry in lymphoma patients treated with radioimmunotherapy. Cancer 2010;116(Suppl 4):1093–100.

10. Buckley SE, Chittenden SJ, Saran FH, et al. Whole-body dosimetry for individualized treatment planning of 131I-MIBG radionuclide therapy for neuroblastoma. J Nucl Med 2009;50(9):1518–24.

11. Flux GD, Haq M, Chittenden SJ, et al. A dose-effect correlation for radioiodine ablation in differentiated thyroid cancer. Eur J Nucl Med Mol Imaging 2010; 37(2):270–5.

12. Shen S, Meredith RF, Duan J, et al. Comparison of methods for predicting myelotoxicity for non-marrow targeting I-131-antibody therapy. Cancer Biother Radiopharm 2003;18(2):209–15.

13. Siegel JA, Yeldell D, Goldenberg DM, et al. Red marrow radiation dose adjustment using plasma FLT3-L cytokine levels: improved correlations between hematologic toxicity and bone marrow dose for radioimmunotherapy patients. J Nucl Med 2003;44(1):67–76.

14. Lassmann M, Reiners C, Luster M. Dosimetry and thyroid cancer: the individual dosage of radioiodine. Endocr Relat Cancer 2010;17(3):R161–72.

15. Sgouros G, Squeri S, Ballangrud ÅM, et al. Non-Hodgkin's lymphoma patients treated with 131 I-anti-B1 antibody: assessment of tumor dose–response. J Nucl Med 2003;44(2):260–8.

16. Prideaux AR, Song H, Hobbs RF, et al. Three-dimensional radiobiologic dosimetry: application of radiobiologic modeling to patient-specific 3-dimensional imaging-based internal dosimetry. J Nucl Med 2007;48(6):1008–16.

17. Sgouros G, Hobbs RF, Atkins FB, et al. Three-dimensional radiobiological dosimetry (3D-RD) with 124I PET for 131I therapy of thyroid cancer. Eur J Nucl Med Mol Imaging 2011;38(Suppl 1): S41–7.

18. Dewaraja YK, Schipper MJ, Roberson PL, et al. 131I-tositumomab radioimmunotherapy: initial tumor dose-response results using 3-dimensional dosimetry including radiobiologic modeling. J Nucl Med 2010;51(7):1155–62.

19. Senthamizhchelvan S, Hobbs RF, Song H, et al. Tumor dosimetry and response for 153Sm-ethylenediamine tetramethylene phosphonic acid therapy of high-risk osteosarcoma. J Nucl Med 2012;53(2):215–24.

20. Dieudonné A, Garin E, Laffont S, et al. Clinical feasibility of fast 3-dimensional dosimetry of the liver for treatment planning of hepatocellular carcinoma with 90Y-microspheres. J Nucl Med 2011; 52(12):1930–7.

21. Cremonesi M, Botta F, Di Dia A, et al. Dosimetry for treatment with radiolabelled somatostatin analogues. A review. Q J Nucl Med Mol Imaging 2010;54(1):37–51.

22. Baechler S, Hobbs RF, Prideaux AR, et al. Extension of the biological effective dose to the MIRD schema and possible implications in radionuclide therapy dosimetry. Med Phys 2008;35(3):1123–34.

23. Wessels BW, Konijnenberg MW, Dale RG, et al. MIRD pamphlet no. 20: the effect of model assumptions on kidney dosimetry and response–implications for radionuclide therapy. J Nucl Med 2008;49(11):1884–99.

24. Kam BL, Teunissen JJ, Krenning EP, et al. Lutetium-labelled peptides for therapy of neuroendocrine tumours. Eur J Nucl Med Mol Imaging 2012; 39(Suppl 1):S103–12.

25. Pauwels S, Barone R. Practical dosimetry of peptide receptor radionuclide therapy with 90 Y-labeled somatostatin analogs. J Nucl Med 2005;46(1):92–8.

26. Barone R, Borson-Chazot F, Valkema R, et al. Patient-specific dosimetry in predicting renal toxicity with (90)Y-DOTATOC: relevance of kidney volume and dose rate in finding a dose-effect relationship. J Nucl Med 2005;46(Suppl 1):99S–106S.

27. Baechler S, Hobbs RF, Boubaker A, et al. Three-dimensional radiobiological dosimetry of kidneys for treatment planning in peptide receptor radionuclide therapy. Med Phys 2012;39(10):6118–28.

28. Schuchardt C, Kulkarni HR, Prasad V, et al. The Bad Berka dose protocol: comparative results of dosimetry in peptide receptor radionuclide therapy using (177)Lu-DOTATATE, (177)Lu-DOTANOC, and (177)Lu-DOTATOC. Recent Results Cancer Res 2013;194:519–36.

29. Remy H, Borget I, Leboulleux S, et al. 131I effective half-life and dosimetry in thyroid cancer patients. J Nucl Med 2008;49(9):1445–50.

30. Forrer F, Uusijärvi H, Waldherr C, et al. A comparison of 111In-DOTATOC and 111In-DOTATATE: biodistribution and dosimetry in the same patients with metastatic neuroendocrine tumours. Eur J Nucl Med Mol Imaging 2004;31(9):1257–62.

31. Barone R, Walrand S, Konijnenberg M, et al. Therapy using labelled somatostatin analogues: comparison of the absorbed doses with 111In-DTPA-D-Phe1-octreotide and yttrium-labelled DOTA-D-Phe1-Tyr3-octreotide. Nucl Med Commun 2008;29(3):283–90.

32. Fabbri C, Sarti G, Cremonesi M, et al. Quantitative analysis of 90Y Bremsstrahlung SPECT-CT images for application to 3D patient-specific dosimetry. Cancer Biother Radiopharm 2009;24(1):145–54.

33. Table of Nuclides. 2002. [Online]. Available at: http://yoyo.cc.monash.edu.au/~simcam/ton/. Accessed 25 May, 2013.

34. Walrand S, Flux GD, Konijnenberg MW, et al. Dosimetry of yttrium-labelled radiopharmaceuticals for internal therapy: 86Y or 90Y imaging? Eur J Nucl Med Mol Imaging 2011;38(Suppl 1):S57–68.

35. Walrand S, Jamar F, Mathieu I, et al. Quantitation in PET using isotopes emitting prompt single gammas: application to yttrium-86. Eur J Nucl Med Mol Imaging 2003;30(3):354–61.

36. Lubberink M, Herzog H. Quantitative imaging of 124I and 86Y with PET. Eur J Nucl Med Mol Imaging 2011;38(Suppl 1):S10–8.

37. Pentlow K, Finn R, Larson S, et al. Quantitative imaging of yttrium-86 with PET. The occurrence and correction of anomalous apparent activity in high density regions. Clin Positron Imaging 2000; 3(3):85–90.

38. Lubberink M, Schneider H, Bergström M, et al. Quantitative imaging and correction for cascade gamma radiation of 76Br with 2D and 3D PET. Phys Med Biol 2002;47(19):3519–34.

39. Herzog H, Tellmann L, Scholten B, et al. PET imaging problems with the non-standard positron emitters yttrium-86 and iodine-124. Q J Nucl Med Mol Imaging 2008;52(2):159–65.

40. Kull T, Ruckgaber J, Weller R, et al. Quantitative imaging of yttrium-86 PET with the ECAT EXACT HR+ in 2D mode. Cancer Biother Radiopharm 2004;19(4):482–90.

41. Beattie BJ, Finn RD, Rowland DJ, et al. Quantitative imaging of bromine-76 and yttrium-86 with PET: a method for the removal of spurious activity introduced by cascade gamma rays. Med Phys 2003; 30(9):2410–23.

42. Flux G, Bardies M, Monsieurs M, et al. The impact of PET and SPECT on dosimetry for targeted radionuclide therapy. Z Med Phys 2006; 16(1):47–59.

43. Zaknun JJ, Bodei L, Mueller-Brand J, et al. The joint IAEA, EANM, and SNMMI practical guidance on peptide receptor radionuclide therapy (PRRNT) in neuroendocrine tumours. Eur J Nucl Med Mol Imaging 2013;40(5):800–16.

44. Lopci E, Chiti A, Castellani MR, et al. Matched pairs dosimetry: 124I/131I metaiodobenzylguanidine

and 124I/131I and 86Y/90Y antibodies. Eur J Nucl Med Mol Imaging 2011;38(Suppl 1):S28–40.

45. Helisch A, Förster GJ, Reber H, et al. Pre-therapeutic dosimetry and biodistribution of 86Y-DOTA-Phe1-Tyr3-octreotide versus 111In-pentetreotide in patients with advanced neuroendocrine tumours. Eur J Nucl Med Mol Imaging 2004;31(10): 1386–92.

46. Förster GJ, Engelbach MJ, Brockmann JJ, et al. Preliminary data on biodistribution and dosimetry for therapy planning of somatostatin receptor positive tumours: comparison of (86)Y-DOTATOC and (111)In-DTPA-octreotide. Eur J Nucl Med 2001; 28(12):1743–50.

47. Jamar F, Barone R, Mathieu I, et al. 86Y-DOTA0)-D-Phe1-Tyr3-octreotide (SMT487)–a phase 1 clinical study: pharmacokinetics, biodistribution and renal protective effect of different regimens of amino acid co-infusion. Eur J Nucl Med Mol Imaging 2003;30(4):510–8.

48. Kappadath S. SU-GG-I-163: a scatter correction algorithm for quantitative yttrium-90 SPECT imaging. Med Phys 2010;37(6):3139.

49. Ito S, Kurosawa H, Kasahara H, et al. (90)Y bremsstrahlung emission computed tomography using gamma cameras. Ann Nucl Med 2009; 23(3):257–67.

50. Minarik D, Ljungberg M, Segars P, et al. Evaluation of quantitative planar 90Y bremsstrahlung whole-body imaging. Phys Med Biol 2009; 54(19):5873–83.

51. Selwyn RG, Nickles RJ, Thomadsen BR, et al. A new internal pair production branching ratio of 90Y: the development of a non-destructive assay for 90Y and 90Sr. Appl Radiat Isot 2007;65(3): 318–27.

52. Nickles RJ, Roberts AD, Nye JA, et al. Assaying and PET imaging of ytrrium-90. IEEE Nucl Sci Symp Conf Rec 2004;6:3412–4.

53. Werner MK, Brechtel K, Beyer T, et al. PET/CT for the assessment and quantification of (90)Y biodistribution after selective internal radiotherapy (SIRT) of liver metastases. Eur J Nucl Med Mol Imaging 2010;37(2):407–8.

54. Gates VL, Esmail AA, Marshall K, et al. Internal pair production of 90Y permits hepatic localization of microspheres using routine PET: proof of concept. J Nucl Med 2011;52(1):72–6.

55. Rault E, Clementel E, Vandenberghe S, et al. Comparison of yttrium-90 SPECT and PET images. J Nucl Med 2010;51(Suppl 2):35.

56. Fabbri C, Mattone V, Casi M, et al. Quantitative evaluation on [90Y] DOTATOC PET and SPECT imaging by phantom acquisitions and clinical applications in locoregional and systemic treatments. Q J Nucl Med Mol Imaging 2012;56(6): 522–8.

57. Lhommel R, Goffette P, Van den Eynde M, et al. Yttrium-90 TOF PET scan demonstrates high-resolution biodistribution after liver SIRT. Eur J Nucl Med Mol Imaging 2009;36(10):1696.

58. Elschot M, Vermolen BJ, Lam MG, et al. Quantitative comparison of PET and bremsstrahlung SPECT for imaging the in vivo yttrium-90 microsphere distribution after liver radioembolization. PLoS One 2013;8(2):e55742.

59. van Elmbt L, Vandenberghe S, Walrand S, et al. Comparison of yttrium-90 quantitative imaging by TOF and non-TOF PET in a phantom of liver selective internal radiotherapy. Phys Med Biol 2011; 56(21):6759–77.

60. Lhommel R, van Elmbt L, Goffette P, et al. Feasibility of 90Y TOF PET-based dosimetry in liver metastasis therapy using SIR-Spheres. Eur J Nucl Med Mol Imaging 2010;37(9):1654–62.

61. Stabin MG, Sparks RB, Crowe E. OLINDA/EXM: the second-generation personal computer software for internal dose assessment in nuclear medicine. J Nucl Med 2005;46(6):1023–7.

62. D'Arienzo M, Chiaramida P, Chiacchiararelli L, et al. 90Y PET-based dosimetry after selective internal radiotherapy treatments. Nucl Med Commun 2012;33(6):633–40.

63. Walrand S, Jamar F, van Elmbt L, et al. 4-Step renal dosimetry dependent on cortex geometry applied to 90Y peptide receptor radiotherapy: evaluation using a fillable kidney phantom imaged by 90Y PET. J Nucl Med 2010;51(12): 1969–73.

64. Bouchet LG, Bolch WE, Blanco HP, et al. MIRD Pamphlet No 19: absorbed fractions and radionuclide S values for six age-dependent multiregion models of the kidney. J Nucl Med 2003;44(7): 1113–47.

65. Rufini V, Baum RP, Castaldi P, et al. Role of PET/CT in the functional imaging of endocrine pancreatic tumors. Abdom Imaging 2012;37(6): 1004–20.

66. Wong KK, Waterfield RT, Marzola MC, et al. Contemporary nuclear medicine imaging of neuroendocrine tumours. Clin Radiol 2012; 67(11):1035–50.

67. Naji M, AL-Nahhas A. 68Ga-labelled peptides in the management of neuroectodermal tumours. Eur J Nucl Med Mol Imaging 2012;39(Suppl 1): S61–7.

68. Ambrosini V, Campana D, Tomassetti P, et al. 68Ga-labelled peptides for diagnosis of gastroenteropancreatic NET. Eur J Nucl Med Mol Imaging 2012;39(Suppl 1):S52–60.

69. Breeman WA, de Blois E, Sze Chan H, et al. (68)Ga-labeled DOTA-peptides and (68)Ga-labeled radiopharmaceuticals for positron emission tomography: current status of research, clinical

applications, and future perspectives. Semin Nucl Med 2011;41(4):314–21.

70. Ezziddin S, Sabet A, Heinemann F, et al. Response and long-term control of bone metastases after peptide receptor radionuclide therapy with (177)Lu-octreotate. J Nucl Med 2011;52(8): 1197–203.

71. Singh B, Prasad V, Schuchardt C, et al. Can the standardized uptake values derived from diagnostic 68 Ga-DOTATATE PET/CT imaging predict the radiation dose delivered to the metastatic liver NET lesions on 177 Lu-DOTATATE peptide receptor radionuclide therapy? J Postgrad Med Educ Res 2013;47:7–13.

72. Scheler S, Fischer R, Fani M, et al. Use of 68Ga-DOTA-TATE PET/CT for predicting the dose of 177Lu-DOTA-TATE therapy in patients with neuroendocrine tumors (NETs). Society Nuclear Medicine Annual Meeting Abstracts 2012; 53(Suppl 1):96.

73. Müller C, Forrer F, Bernard BF, et al. Diagnostic versus therapeutic doses of [(177)Lu-DOTA-Tyr(3)]-octreotate: uptake and dosimetry in somatostatin receptor-positive tumors and normal organs. Cancer Biother Radiopharm 2007;22(1):151–9.

74. Koumarianou E, Loktionova NS, Fellner M, et al. 44Sc-DOTA-BN[2-14]NH2 in comparison to 68Ga-DOTA-BN[2-14]NH2 in pre-clinical investigation. Is 44Sc a potential radionuclide for PET? Appl Radiat Isot 2012;70(12):2669–76.

75. Rösch F, Baum RP. Generator-based PET radiopharmaceuticals for molecular imaging of tumours: on the way to THERANOSTICS. Dalton Trans 2011; 40(23):6104–11.

76. Walrand S, Barone R, Pauwels S, et al. Experimental facts supporting a red marrow uptake due to radiometal transchelation in 90Y-DOTATOC therapy and relationship to the decrease of platelet counts. Eur J Nucl Med Mol Imaging 2011;38(7): 1270–80.

# Index

*Note:* Page numbers of article titles are in **boldface** type.

PET Clin 9 (2014) 113–115
http://dx.doi.org/10.1016/S1556-8598(13)00120-X
1556-8598/14/$ – see front matter © 2014 Elsevier Inc. All rights reserved.

# Moving?

## Make sure your subscription moves with you!

To notify us of your new address, find your **Clinics Account Number** (located on your mailing label above your name), and contact customer service at:

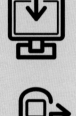

**Email: journalscustomerservice-usa@elsevier.com**

**800-654-2452** (subscribers in the U.S. & Canada)
**314-447-8871** (subscribers outside of the U.S. & Canada)

**Fax number: 314-447-8029**

**Elsevier Health Sciences Division**
**Subscription Customer Service**
**3251 Riverport Lane**
**Maryland Heights, MO 63043**

*To ensure uninterrupted delivery of your subscription, please notify us at least 4 weeks in advance of move.

ELSEVIER